Have A Magnificent Menopause:

A Straightforward Guide to Looking Good and Feeling Great

ALISON BLADH

C Published in 2025 by Discover Your Bounce Publishing
www.discoveryourbouncepublishing.com
Copyright © Discover Your Bounce Publishing
All rights reserved.

ISBN: 978-1-914428-36-4

Although the author and publisher have made every effort to ensure that the
information in this book is correct at the time of going to print, the author
and publisher do not assume and therefore disclaim liability to any party. The
author and the publisher will not be held responsible for any loss or damage
save for that caused by their negligence.

Although the author and the publisher have made every reasonable attempt to
achieve accuracy in the content of this book, they assume no responsibility for
errors or omissions.

Page design and typesetting by Discover Your Bounce Publishing
copyright © 2025 Alison Bladh

DEDICATION

To all the women in my life, past, present and still to come.
To my mother, who left far too soon but whose love lives on in
everything I do. I would be nothing without you all.
This book is for you.

Praise for Have a Magnificent Menopause

"Alison Bladh has shared her wisdom with an incredible and pragmatic way to help all of us going through the transition from perimenopause, menopause and post menopause. Have a Magnificent Menopause is a reflection of Alison's exceptional expertise as a Nutritionist and Counselor using diet as medicine. I heartily recommend this to all women who want to keep living their best life"

Gerianne DiPiano -
Founder & CEO Of Femme Pharma Consumer Healthcare

"Fabulous book, like having your own menopause mentor in your pocket. Packed with science backed information, health hacks and compassionate support"

Sara Andrews BA (Hons), PGDip TA Psychotherapy, NCPS Accred. - Psychotherapeutic Counsellor & Mind Shift Coach

"Have a Magnificent Menopause is an informative and reassuring book that offers both knowledge and hope to women during a life phase often met with silence. Alison Bladh writes with empathy, humour and scientific clarity, making it easy to absorb both the facts and practical advice. More than just a guide to menopause, it's an inspiring reminder that this time of life can mark a powerful new beginning. Highly recommended for all women and their loved ones."

Mariana Holmberg -
50, a busy professional on a mission to feel good again

"Working with Alison changed everything for me and this book feels just like having her right beside you. It's filled with the same practical, caring advice that helped me regain my energy, lose weight and feel confident in myself again."

Kirsten J 51 - One of Alison's clients, now thriving through menopause

"Have a Magnificent Menopause is an insightful and practical guide for women navigating perimenopause, menopause and beyond. Alison Bladh's unique dual expertise in nutritional therapy and beauty therapy offers a compassionate, science-backed approach that supports women both physically and emotionally, including those who cannot or choose not to use HRT. A must-read for women who feel overwhelmed or unheard, this book is a powerful reminder that menopause can be a magnificent journey."

Erika Ferreira BA, MSc. CIDESCO - Global Head of Marketing, Author.

"As someone who speaks to women every day about menopause, ageing, confidence and self-worth, this book is a breath of fresh air. A roadmap to feeling good. She strips away the shame and gives us permission to feel fabulous again. Alison gets it, and every page shows it."

Lisa Nash - TV Presenter and Podcaster

"A straightforward approach that is easy to follow and produces extraordinary results.

There is a lot of information available about navigating through the years of menopause but this book brings it all together with an easy to implement approach which really works. Alison explains the science around the 'why', invaluable for every woman who is struggling to understand the changes that are taking place in her body.

Alison's straightforward approach is suitable for every woman whether she is taking HRT or like me unable to use traditional HRT to manage the distressing symptoms.

Alison's nutrition advice uses food as medicine and also explains how small behavioural changes can make a huge difference in managing symptoms as well as the latest developments in the beauty industry to truly make the most of this time in a woman's life. She busts the myth that it is impossible to lose weight during the menopause.

Alison's advice is easy to follow and produces extraordinary results. I am happier, healthier, glowing and full of energy and am now the same weight as I was in my 30's!"

Carolyn Hicks - 59, Menopause Warrior

"This book is exactly what I needed. It's honest, practical and gave me real answers. I feel more like me again. Every woman over 40 should read it."

Rachel Thomas - 52, working mum finally putting herself first

CONTENTS

ACKNOWLEDGEMENTS

Thank you to the clients who have shared their stories with me, your honesty, resilience and experiences have shaped every chapter of this book.

To my colleagues, mentors and the professionals who have challenged and supported me, your insight and encouragement have been truly invaluable.

To Discover Your Bounce, your support, guidance and belief in me helped bring this book to life.

And to my family and friends, thank you for your unwavering love, patience and belief in me throughout this journey.

HOW TO USE THIS BOOK

This book is here for you to use however you need it. You don't have to read it from start to finish, though I hope you will. Feel free to dip in and out, choosing the chapters that resonate with you most.

It's a practical, hands-on, action-based guide designed to support you through the ups and downs of this stage in life. Come back to it whenever you're having a rough day or need extra help. Whether you're looking for a quick tip, a reminder to prioritise yourself, a plan to get back on track, or a beauty boost, this book is your trusted no-nonsense companion for feeling and looking your best.

For simplicity, throughout this book, I use the term menopause to refer to the entire transition including perimenopause, menopause and postmenopause. I do this to keep things easy to read and avoid repetition, but know that everything I share is relevant no matter which stage you're in.

A NOTE ON SUPPLEMENTS IN THIS BOOK

Throughout this book, you'll find supplement suggestions at the end of some chapters. In my practice, I always take a food-first approach because real, nourishing food is the foundation of good health. However, supplements can have a place, especially during perimenopause and menopause, when your body may need extra support.

That said, supplements should be treated with respect. They can interact with medications or affect underlying health conditions. Always speak with your doctor or a qualified practitioner before starting anything new.

Please avoid buying supplements from the supermarket or online bargain shops. These are often low in potency and contain nutrients in poorly absorbed forms which is why they're cheap. When possible, choose practitioner-quality products or buy from your local independent health food shop, where you can ask for guidance and trust the quality.

INTRODUCTION

Have you ever looked in the mirror, feeling exhausted and wondered if you'll ever feel like yourself again? Balanced, energised and gently confident in both how you look and feel? Or maybe you're fed up of looking in your wardrobe, frustrated that nothing fits the woman staring back at you. Perhaps you're questioning why you're always so tired, irritable, sad or why you've lost your love for life. If any of this sounds familiar, take a deep breath. You've found me (and my book!) and I understand exactly how you feel and where you are right now.

My mission is simple: I want every woman to feel incredible in her own skin. To have that feeling of walking into a room, head held high, heels clicking, feeling fabulous and full of life. That energy doesn't need to disappear after 40. Perimenopause and menopause are transitions, not endings and postmenopause is a powerful new chapter. Together, we're going to explore how to keep that inner vibrancy alive and let the world know, "I'm still here and I'm full of life."

Let's be honest while we all want to feel better, many of us also want to look good. It's the thing so many women feel they shouldn't say out loud, as if wanting to look your best is somehow less valid than focusing on your health. I'm here to say what everyone's thinking but feels they can't say: it's OK to want both.

In fact, the two go hand in hand. When you feel good, you often look better and when you like what you see in the mirror, it can boost your confidence and make you feel amazing. Taking care of yourself, whether it's through skincare, healthy eating, exercise or professional treatments, isn't vanity it's self-care.

The feedback I've received from the many women I have had the pleasure of working with has been clear, they appreciate someone finally saying it. Because yes, this is about feeling better, but it's also about looking as vibrant and fabulous as you are at every stage of life. And that's nothing to feel guilty about.

In my 35 years of working with women in this stage of life, I've seen the power of approaching health holistically using lifestyle medicine. I know personally what it's like to feel lost in the noise of different health solutions that don't quite fit. Today, there is a lot of focus on HRT and while it's wonderful that this conversation is finally happening, it can feel isolating for those of us who, like myself, can't take it, or those who choose not to. Women like us can feel overlooked, worrying we'll be left to struggle through symptoms with nothing but vague advice.

For these women, it can be a lonely place. Without other options in sight, there's a genuine fear of being left to battle with symptoms, feeling like we're on a steady decline. But don't worry because you are not alone! I've seen the incredible transformation that lifestyle-based wellness can bring. Nutrition, daily routines, mindset shifts, and beauty practices can offer a pathway to inner and outer radiance, all with or without HRT. Women's lives at this stage are far richer and more complex than anything that can be resolved with pills, patches, or gels alone.

Let me share a bit of my story. I've been passionate about skincare and wellness ever since I was a teenager battling acne. Even back then, I was driven to understand why my skin was reacting that way and what I could do about it. I experimented with diet and made small lifestyle tweaks that, to my amazement, eventually made a difference. That early experience sparked my career as a beauty therapist, where I began to see firsthand how transformative skincare, aesthetic treatments, mindset and nutrition could be. But it was my love of understanding hormones and their profound impact on the body that led me to work with women going through menopause.

More and more, I attracted clients in these stages of life who were struggling not only with their skin but with energy, weight, mood swings and a deep sense of feeling lost in their own bodies. Listening to their stories, I quickly realised how neglected many of these women felt, how often they were brushed off and how debilitating the symptoms of menopause could be. I heard about their daily battles, the exhaustion, the brain fog, skin changes and the intense emotions.

I had seen this before. I remember sitting with my wonderful mother and her friends, listening to them talk about what they were going through. They laughed and shared stories, but beneath it all lingered the unspoken truth, this was something they simply had to endure. They had no support, no real guidance and certainly no conversation about solutions. It struck me even then how unfair it was that women were left to figure it all out on their own, to quietly suffer through changes that impacted every part of their lives.

This understanding ignited a desire in me to go even deeper. I returned to university to study nutritional therapy and lifestyle medicine. Using functional medicine, I gained a deeper understanding of how the right foods, lifestyle shifts, mindset and holistic approaches can profoundly change our well-being. Working with women over 40, I witnessed time and again how skin health, energy and emotional balance are so intricately connected to what's happening inside us.

Having experienced (and still am) menopause this book is my lived experience, a way of bringing that knowledge and experience to you. It's not just a guide; it's a supportive companion on your journey, helping you reclaim a sense of strength, beauty, and wellness that's uniquely yours. This book is about giving you choices; a health and beauty hamper of evidence-based practices that work, whether you're on HRT or not. It's about empowerment, about celebrating the beauty, strength and vitality within us at every stage. There's no one-size-fits-all answer and there's no 'right' or 'wrong' way to approach menopause only what's right for you.

And let's be honest, wanting to look good as we age is a perfectly human desire. It might not always be at the top of your priorities, especially when dealing with other menopausal symptoms, but feeling good about how we look can significantly impact our confidence and overall well-being. It's not vain to want to preserve what we've got as we age; it's a natural and healthy part of self-care. Embracing our beauty at every age and stage helps us feel confident and fulfilled. This book is here to remind you that you can look and feel fabulous, no matter where you are on this journey.

After talking with many women about what they'd like in a book like this, I knew it needed to be easy to read, with actionable advice. One woman said to me just cut the crap and tell me what to do! I believe every woman has the right to feel and look amazing and I know it's crucial you don't feel overwhelmed by loads of hard to digest information. Brain fog, exhaustion and lack of focus are real challenges, so each chapter is designed with simple, easy to read practical steps and insights you can use right away.

Remember, it's not all about menopause. We can't blame everything on good old menopause. Yes, menopause brings unique changes, but we also have the natural ageing process at work. So, if you're ready to explore natural ways to support yourself as you age and transition through menopause let's begin. I hope this book becomes a resource you can dip into whenever you need a boost, a strategy, or a moment of encouragement. You're not alone and with the right approach, this new phase of life can be one of strength, confidence, happiness and vibrant health.

I've seen countless women in my clinic feel just like you do at this moment. I've seen what works. Now, let me show you how it can work for you too.

1 THE MENOPAUSE PUZZLE -
UNDERSTAND WHAT'S HAPPENING INSIDE YOU

"Just when the caterpillar thought the world was over,
it became a butterfly."

Anonymous

Five Things You'll Learn in this Chapter:

- **Knowledge is Power**. Understanding what's happening in your body demystifies the emotional and physical shifts, giving you back a sense of control.

- **The Three-Phase Journey**. Menopause includes perimenopause, menopause and post-menopause each with its own changes and needs.

- **An Evolutionary Gift**. The Grandmother Hypothesis shows menopause as a strength, a time to lead, guide and support future generations.

- **Daily Habits Matter**. Hormones drive the change, but your lifestyle, from sleep to hydration, shapes your experience.

- **Don't Fall for the Hype**. Ignore the myths and marketing. Focus on real, evidence-based solutions.

Menopause can often feel like a mystery, creeping up slowly and suddenly throwing you into a whirlwind of symptoms. From hot flushes and exhaustion to night sweats and unexpected changes in your skin and hair, it can leave you looking in the mirror and wondering, "What on earth happened to me?

It's no wonder menopause feels like such a mystery, especially when so many of us are left in the dark about what to expect. Growing up, no one really talked about it. For many women, it's only when symptoms start to show up that they realise they've entered this new phase of life.

Interestingly, the word "menopause" was first introduced by French doctor Charles Pierre Louis de Gardanne in his book *De La Ménopause Ou De L'âge Critique Des Femmes (The Critical Age of a Woman)*. If you're curious, it's still available on Amazon though I doubt it will answer all your questions! The word itself comes from the Greek *pausis* (pause) and *mēn* (month), which, let's be honest, is a bit underwhelming for what we're actually going through.

Thankfully, the narrative is shifting. I love the new terms women are using to redefine this stage, like "queenagers" or "fabsters." These are such positive, empowering words and frankly, I'd much rather be called a "fabster" than "menopausal."

But let's not sugar-coat it: menopause is intense. It's a time that can make you feel like you're at breaking point, exhausted, overwhelmed and desperate for relief.

Here's the good news: menopause isn't just random chaos, even though it might feel that way. There are real, physical reasons behind the changes in your body. The more you understand what's happening, the more empowered you'll feel to take back control. Knowledge really is power, it's the key to reclaiming your body, looks, mind and sense of well-being.

> The more you understand, the more in control you'll feel.

Knowledge isn't just power, it's your key to taking charge of your body, your health and how you feel every single day.

In this chapter, we'll explore what's really happening inside you. You don't need to become a hormone expert; I'll break it all down in a way that's clear and practical. By the end, you'll feel more at ease, more in control and ready to take the first steps towards feeling and looking like yourself again.

The Hormonal Rollercoaster – What's Really Happening

There are three big hormonal events in a woman's life. Puberty, a well-known and frequently discussed hormonal event, which brings about a sudden influx of hormones leading to many changes that can sometimes cause the typical teenage turbulence and mood swings! Pregnancy is another major hormonal event in a woman's life that we commonly talk about. And then there's the menopause which tends to be shrouded in silence! It's the silent transition that every woman will go through, but we rarely speak about. Menopause is like an unexpected guest who shows up to your house unannounced, stays indefinitely and unpacks all her bags.

Before I get started, let's take a moment to recap how it all works. We get our first period during puberty a phase most of us remember all too well. Then, years later, comes what many call the second puberty, perimenopause. And honestly, as if one rollercoaster wasn't enough, we're faced with another round of hormonal ups and downs. This time, though, it often feels even more unpredictable.

From puberty onwards, a group of hormones work together to regulate the menstrual cycle, which typically lasts around 21 to 35 days, with an average of 28 days. During the first half of the cycle, oestrogen rises, thickening the lining of the womb in preparation for pregnancy. Around the middle of the cycle, typically between days 12 and 16 in a 28-day cycle ovulation occurs, releasing an egg from the ovary.

Progesterone works with oestrogen to prepare the womb for pregnancy. If no fertilisation occurs, hormone levels fall, the lining breaks down, and menstruation begins and the cycle starts again.

Known as the "calming hormone," progesterone regulates your menstrual cycle, supports pregnancy, promotes restful sleep, reduces anxiety and helps balance mood.

Fig.1 The Hormonal Cycle

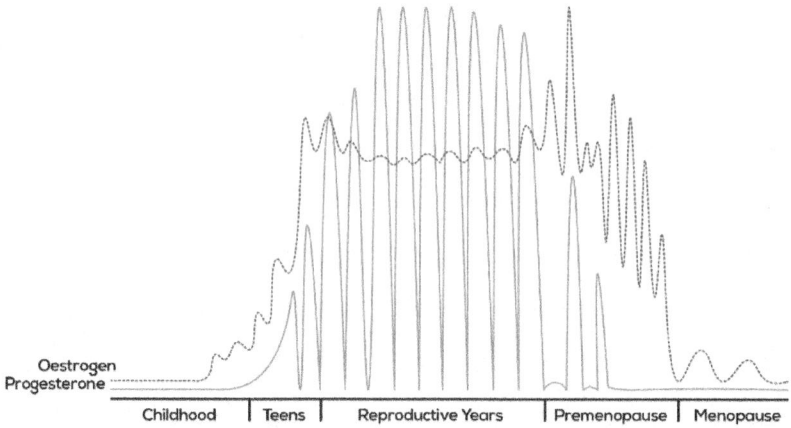

| Childhood | Teens | Reproductive Years | Premenopause | Menopause |

Oestrogen and progesterone work in harmony to regulate your cycle, but during menopause, this balance shifts.

When we approach menopause, the production of these hormones starts to gradually decline. This causes periods to become irregular and eventually they will stop completely. This process can take many years. The process that we go through is called the menopause transition, which consists of three phases.

Perimenopause: The average age for perimenopause is 45. Think of this as the warm-up before menopause, usually starting in your 40s. Of course, this can vary depending on where you live in the world, as lifestyle, ethnicity, socioeconomic status, environmental conditions, genetics and overall health all play a role. During this time, hormone levels start to fluctuate wildly and can become unbalanced. You might notice changes like irregular or heavy periods, mood swings, weight gain, fatigue, or even those famous hot flushes. This phase can last for several years or more.

Menopause: This is the milestone, often around age 51. When you haven't had a period for 12 months consecutively, you are officially in the menopause. You might not have had a period for 10 months and you are well on your way to menopause, but then you get one, which means you are still in perimenopause waiting at the menopause door to be let in. During this time, hormone levels drop significantly and symptoms like hot flushes and sleep disruptions can get worse. It can feel intense and exhausting.

Post-menopause: This is all the time after menopause, which is the rest of your life which can be 30 years plus as we are living longer. Some symptoms might ease up slowly, but lower hormone levels can increase your risk for chronic diseases like osteoporosis, heart disease and cognitive decline. It's more important than ever to focus on self-care and prevention to stay healthy, happy and strong.

Testosterone: The Forgotten Hormone in Menopause

We often hear about oestrogen and progesterone during menopause, but testosterone is another hormone that plays an important role in our health and well-being. While we typically associate testosterone with men, women also produce this hormone, though in smaller amounts. Testosterone helps maintain muscle mass, bone density, energy levels, cognitive health and even influences our sexual desire, which can dwindle as we age. As we move through the menopause transition, testosterone levels also decline. This is not directly related to the menopause, as testosterone levels decline gradually as we age. Some women opt to take testosterone hormone therapy though current evidence only supports its use for persistent low libido. .Accessing treatment can be challenging and it's not always available through your healthcare provider. It's important to discuss your options thoroughly with your doctor to determine what's right for you.

Oestrogen, the key female hormone, regulates everything from reproduction to mood and bone health. With receptors in the brain, heart, skin and bones it has an impact on virtually every function in the body.

The Wisdom of Menopause:
Lessons from Nature's Matriarchs

Did you know that humans aren't the only ones to experience menopause? It's a rare phenomenon shared by only a few species on Earth, placing us among an extraordinary group. Alongside us, only a handful of animals including the majestic killer whales, beluga whales and short-finned pilot whales undergo menopause. These remarkable creatures stop reproducing halfway through their lives yet continue to play vital roles within their social groups, much like we do as we become grandparents, mentors, leaders and sources of strength within our communities.

Some of us guide younger generations in the workplace, while others become pillars of support for friends, volunteers, advocates, or the glue that holds families together in different ways. Whether through caregiving, leadership, friendship, or making an impact in the world around us, our value doesn't diminish it evolves.

Menopause isn't about fading into the background or becoming less relevant. It's about stepping into a new kind of power one where experience, wisdom and purpose shape the next chapter of our lives in ways that extend far beyond motherhood.

Imagine a pod of killer whales gliding through the ocean, led by an older female who no longer reproduces but whose wisdom is essential for survival. She knows where to find food, senses danger before it arrives and ensures the safety of her pod. She is their guide, their protector, their source of knowledge. Menopause doesn't weaken her; it strengthens her role.

Did you know humans aren't the only species to experience menopause? Killer whales, beluga whales and short-finned pilot whales also go through this unique transition. These magnificent creatures stop reproducing and take on roles in the pod as wise leaders, guiding and protecting their families.

For us, this transition isn't about what's ending; it's about stepping into a different kind of guardianship. We become the steady hand that others look to, the voice of experience that provides reassurance and the presence that holds everything together. This idea, known as the Grandmother Hypothesis, suggests that older, non-reproductive women have been a vital evolutionary advantage for humanity passing down wisdom, nurturing future generations, and shaping the survival of families and societies.

Menopause, then, isn't a flaw of nature. It's an evolutionary gift. Just like the powerful whale matriarchs leading their pods through unknown waters, we guide our families, our communities and ourselves through life's ever-changing tides. This stage of life isn't about decline; it's about stepping into our fullest, strongest and most invaluable role yet.

Early Menopause and Primary Ovarian Insufficiency (POI)

Menopause is commonly associated with women in their late 40s and early 50s, but for some, it arrives much earlier. Experiencing menopause before the age of 45 is considered early menopause and for some women, it can happen even before they turn 40 due to a condition called Premature Ovarian Insufficiency (POI).

POI occurs when the ovaries stop functioning properly before the age of 40, leading to irregular or absent periods, fertility issues and symptoms of low oestrogen such as hot flushes, night sweats, fatigue and mood changes. Unlike natural menopause, where hormone levels decline gradually, in most cases of POI this decline is also gradual, but it can be sudden if caused by medical treatment or surgical menopause.

What Causes Early Menopause?

There are several reasons why some women experience menopause earlier than expected:

Premature Ovarian Insufficiency (POI): A condition where the ovaries stop working properly before age 40.

Genetics: If your mother or grandmother went through menopause early, you may have a higher chance of experiencing it too.

Medical Treatments: Cancer treatments like chemotherapy or radiation can damage ovarian function and trigger early menopause.

Surgery: Removal of the ovaries (oophorectomy) leads to immediate menopause, known as surgical menopause, which can bring on more severe symptoms.

Autoimmune Conditions: Certain autoimmune diseases, like thyroid disorders, lupus, or Addison's disease, can affect ovarian function.

Think of oestrogen like your body's thermostat. When it's working properly, you stay nice and comfortable. But when it starts to malfunction, things can suddenly get really hot!
Say hello to the hot flush!

Why It's Important to Recognise Early Menopause

Experiencing menopause early can be extremely physically and emotionally challenging, especially if you're not expecting it. Early menopause can increase the risk of osteoporosis, heart disease and cognitive decline due to the long-term effects of low oestrogen. Women in this situation may also struggle with fertility concerns or feel isolated because menopause isn't typically associated with younger women.

If you suspect you might be going through menopause earlier than expected, it's important to speak to a doctor and explore hormone therapy (HRT) and lifestyle changes that can support your health.

You're not alone, and there are ways to manage this transition so you can still feel your best. There are resources at the back of this book to help you.

Spotting the Signs. Symptoms of Menopause

The symptoms of menopause form a long and varied list and every woman's experience is unique. Some glide through menopause with barely a change, while for others, symptoms range from mild to completely debilitating.

One of the most prevalent symptoms is joint and muscular pain, according to a comprehensive meta-analysis involving 482,067 women worldwide. The study found that 65.43% of participants experienced this discomfort. In Europe, additional research revealed that 70% of women reported night sweats, while 79% experienced hot flushes. Cognitive symptoms were also common, with 20% struggling with memory issues, brain fog and difficulty concentrating, while 18% experienced unexpected joint pain, and 22% suffered from sleeping problems or insomnia.

Have you ever heard of formication? It's one of those strange and lesser-known menopause symptoms, a sensation that feels like insects crawling on your skin. Many women suffer from it without realising it's linked to hormonal changes.

Menopause is very real and it affects women in different ways across the world. These symptoms, though frustrating, are a natural part of this transition even when they don't feel like it. If you find yourself suddenly feeling more irritable, waking up drenched in sweat, or struggling to focus, it could be a sign that your body is shifting into this new phase.

Beyond the internal changes, menopause can also affect how you look. You might notice dark circles and puffiness under your eyes from poor sleep, dry and itchy skin, pigmentation marks on your face and hands and even hair thinning or hair loss. Oh, and just when you thought you'd had enough surprises, your lip volume can shrink by up to 60%!. These changes can be frustrating and may knock your confidence, making you feel unlike yourself but understanding them is the first step in taking back control. These changes can be really distressing and may knock your confidence, making you feel unlike yourself.

But here's what you need to know: you are not alone and you are not powerless. Understanding these changes is the first step in taking back control.

Up to 79% of women experience hot flushes during menopause, but symptoms can vary greatly from insomnia to joint pain.

No two journeys are exactly alike.

Which Symptoms are Showing Up for You?

Symptoms of perimenopause and menopause often subtly sneak into our lives, making it easy to dismiss them or attribute them to life in general or just getting older. Many of the women I work with are genuinely surprised when I explain that their symptoms whether physical, emotional, or mental could be linked to menopause.

"Overwhelmed by exhaustion and unsure where to start? Small, practical changes can transform how you feel and look, helping you regain energy, confidence and radiant skin even when life feels chaotic."

Client story

One of my clients, (Sarah, 46 years old), came to me feeling completely exhausted and overwhelmed. She described how her energy had plummeted, her mood was unpredictable and she had started waking up in the middle of the night sweating. On top of that, she noticed her skin was drier than before and she was suffering from hair loss. All these things had really started to affect her confidence and she wasn't as happy as she normally would be. She assumed it was just the stresses of everyday life catching up with her or perhaps a lingering health issue she hadn't figured out. When I mentioned these could be symptoms of perimenopause, she was shocked. It hadn't even crossed her mind that her body was transitioning into this phase of life. It was a light bulb moment for her and suddenly, things started to make sense. When she realised her body was experiencing these symptoms because of the hormonal imbalances of perimenopause, this brought her a sense of relief. She wasn't 'falling apart', her body was just telling her it was time for a new approach to her health and well-being

Now that we've explored the hormonal changes and the symptoms they can bring, let's shift our focus to something equally important: how our lifestyle and daily habits influence the way we feel. While hormones play a significant role, they're not the whole story, our choices and routines have a powerful impact too.

It's Not Just About Hormones

Fig.2 Lifestyle Balance

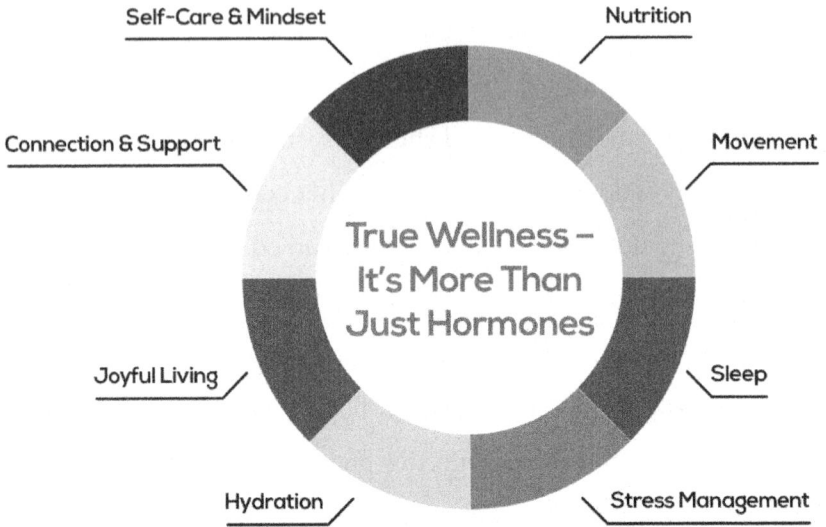

Self-Care & Mindset · Nutrition · Connection & Support · Movement · Joyful Living · Sleep · Hydration · Stress Management

True Wellness – It's More Than Just Hormones

Hormones may drive the changes we experience during menopause, but how we live our daily lives shapes how we feel. This transition is a wake-up call, a reminder that we need to take better care of ourselves.

I have my 80/20 rule that I use with my clients: if you do everything right 80% of the time; you have 20% to enjoy life's little pleasures, a glass of wine, a few chocolate chip biscuits, or whatever makes you happy. But during menopause, that balance shifts. The 80/20 rule becomes 90/10 because our bodies need more support. That doesn't mean giving up everything you love, it simply means making more mindful choices. And don't worry, that 10% still allows room for joy, just in moderation.

> Hormones drive change, but daily habits shape how we experience menopause. It's time to put yourself first!

Small Choices, Big Impact

Menopause isn't just about hormones, it's about the daily habits that either calm the storm or stir it up. The way we eat, move, manage stress and rest all impact how we feel. A diet high in sugar can worsen joint pain and hot flushes, dehydration can amplify brain fog and stress can intensify weight gain and anxiety.

Yet, life at this stage is already relentless balancing careers, managing a household, supporting teenage children who still need you and often caring for ageing parents at the same time. There's never enough time, never enough energy and always someone who needs something from you. Many women in their 40s and beyond feel utterly drained, constantly pulled in different directions, and running on an empty tank, with no chance to refuel.

Then menopause hits. The brain fog, exhaustion, mood swings and sleep struggles pile on top of everything else, making even the simplest tasks feel overwhelming. Add hormonal changes into the mix and suddenly it's like trying to climb a mountain with no map, no rest stops and no end in sight.

I see so many of my clients at the end of their tether, unsure where to turn. That's exactly why I wrote this book: to offer simple, sustainable and realistic ways to integrate meaningful changes into your daily life changes that will truly make a difference.

I know you don't have time to overhaul your entire lifestyle or completely reinvent your nutrition. But even small, daily changes can have a profound impact on your energy, mood and overall well-being.

Your Skin: The Mirror of Your Well-Being

When you're exhausted or overwhelmed, appearance may not seem like a priority. But your skin, nails and hair are often the first to show the effects of your lifestyle choices.

Hormonal changes can leave skin drier, thinner, less elastic, and more prone to fine lines, wrinkles, pigmentation, irritation and even acne! Some women notice uneven skin tone, dark circles, or redness seemingly overnight. It's frustrating, but the good news is you have more control than you think.

Your daily habits play a powerful role in how your skin looks and feels. Staying hydrated, eating nutrient-dense foods, using quality skincare products, managing stress and getting quality sleep can bring back your glow. Even small tweaks like protecting your skin from the sun or establishing a consistent skincare routine can make a visible difference.

With the right care, you can feel confident in your skin, no matter what changes come your way.

Quick Win: Hydration Boost

Start your day with a big glass of warm water before anything else. Staying hydrated supports energy, brain function and skin health. A simple habit that sets a positive tone for the day.

Thriving, Not Just Surviving

As we move through menopause, it becomes clear that hormones may shape the transition, but our lifestyle choices determine how we experience it. Managing stress, staying active and nourishing your body with delicious, nutrient-rich foods are powerful tools for thriving.

Every small change builds momentum, helping you feel and look your best one small step at a time.

Myth-Busting –
Debunking Menopause Misconceptions

Menopause, though more openly discussed in some countries today, is still stigmatised as something negative. Growing up in a strict British household, I remember watching my mother and the women around her, all navigating perimenopause, suffering through what was then simply referred to as "The Change." Nobody talked about it. It was shrouded in silence, misconceptions and misinformation.

While things are improving slowly in some parts of the world, this isn't the case everywhere and there's still a lot of work to be done. Women deserve knowledge, support and care during this natural stage of life.

Not so long ago, in the Victorian era, menopause was associated with something called "climacteric insanity" a term that reflected society's complete misunderstanding of this transition. If a woman showed signs of menopause, such as irritability or mood swings (like shouting at her husband!), she might be labelled as mentally unstable. The 'solution'? Confinement in asylums, where many women were subjected to cruel and dehumanising treatment, often restrained or dismissed as hysterical. The prevailing belief at the time was that the womb influenced the brain, leaving women supposedly more prone to madness.

Thankfully, we've come a long way since then! Medical science has debunked such damaging notions and we now have a far better understanding of menopause as a natural transition. But there's still a lingering sense of shame or embarrassment attached to it, making it harder for many women to seek the help they need.

In some parts of the world, menopause awareness has increased significantly. Everyone seems to be jumping on the bandwagon, which has led to more conversations and available resources for women. This is a positive shift, without a doubt. However, with this rise in awareness has come a flood of misinformation, often in the form of 'menowashing'.

'Menowashing' refers to the growing trend of brands and influencers' marketing products and services as essential for menopause, often without scientific evidence to back up their claims. While some of these products might be genuinely helpful, many are simply cashing in on women's vulnerabilities, offering quick fixes that promise the world but deliver very little. This surge of misleading information can leave women feeling confused and unsure about what's truly effective.

It's more important than ever to focus on evidence-based solutions and reliable advice. Many of the claims being made from miracle supplements to unnecessary treatments lack proper research or validation. That's why I'm passionate about cutting through the noise and providing accurate, practical guidance to help you make informed decisions during this transition.

So, let's bust some of the most common myths I hear in my practice, like "weight gain is inevitable" or "menopause marks the end of your sex life" so you can approach this time of life with clarity and confidence.

Myth vs Truth

Myth	Truth
Menopause always comes with severe symptoms.	Not every woman experiences severe symptoms. Some may have mild or no symptoms at all and these symptoms are very individual and can vary widely.
Weight Gain is inevitable during menopause.	Weight gain during menopause is quite common due to hormonal changes, but it's not inevitable. Lifestyle changes, balanced nutrition, mindset and regular movement can help manage weight effectively.

Menopause only affects your reproductive health.	Menopause affects more than just reproductive health; it can affect brain function, bone health, cardiovascular health, metabolic health and the skin. It really is a whole-body experience.
Hormone Replacement Therapy (HRT) is dangerous.	HRT isn't inherently dangerous; for many women, it can significantly help ease symptoms. Individual health factors determine the safety of HRT and you should always discuss it with a healthcare provider to determine the best course of action.
Hot flushes are the only symptom of menopause.	Menopause has over 40 symptoms, including night sweats, mood swings, weight gain, depression, fatigue, brain fog, dry skin and joint pain. Hot flushes are quite common, but certainly not the only challenge.
Menopause means the end of sexual desire.	While a decrease in libido is an issue for some women, it's far from inevitable. With the right physical care, emotional support and open communication, many

	women continue to enjoy a fulfilling and satisfying sex life during and well beyond, menopause.
Natural strategies don't work for menopause.	Natural approaches, such as dietary changes, mindfulness, exercise, lifestyle modifications and certain supplements, can significantly help manage symptoms. These can work well on their own or alongside medical options like HRT.
Menopause makes you seem older and less attractive.	Menopause does not mean losing your beauty. Self-care, nutrition, quality skincare products, beauty therapy and lifestyle adjustments help maintain healthy, glowing skin and appearance.
You can't build muscle or stay fit after menopause.	While hormonal changes can make it harder to maintain muscle mass and strength, it's far from impossible. Resistance training, strength exercises, and adequate protein intake are powerful tools to help maintain muscle, boost metabolism, and keep your body strong well into

	your 50s, 60s and beyond.
Your skin and hair will never be the same.	Yes, hormonal changes can lead to thinner hair, drier skin and more fine lines, but that doesn't mean you can't have healthy, glowing skin and strong hair. Nutrient-rich foods, collagen support, hydration, scalp care, and targeted beauty treatments can make a real difference in maintaining your hair and skin health during and after menopause.
Menopause turns you into a forgetful mess.	Okay, so you might walk into a room and forget why you're there, but let's be honest, wasn't that happening before menopause too? While brain fog is real, it's not permanent. Exercise, good nutrition, quality sleep, and mental stimulation can all help keep your brain sharp. So, if you've ever spent five minutes looking for your glasses when they were on your head the whole time, don't worry, you're are not alone!

We've now started to peel back the layers of what's really happening inside your body during menopause. Understanding that you are not crazy and that your hormones have an effect on virtually all bodily systems. The next chapters will equip you with the tools you need to take charge and improve your inner and outer well-being. For now, just remember menopause doesn't have to be a mystery. You have more power than you think!

Expanding the Menopause Conversation

While this book is written for women over 40, it's important to acknowledge that menopause isn't exclusive to cisgender women. Transgender men and non-binary people who have ovaries can also experience menopause whether naturally or as a result of medical treatment. Their experience may be different and often more complex, so inclusive support and understanding is essential for everyone going through this life stage.

It's also important to recognise that menopause affects people differently based on many factors, including ethnicity, genetics, socioeconomic background, environmental exposures, disability, neurodiversity and access to care. For example, research suggests that Black women may experience more intense and longer-lasting hot flushes, while some Asian women report fewer vasomotor symptoms but more joint pain. Women with ADHD or other forms of neurodivergence may find their symptoms, such as overwhelm or brain fog, worsen with hormonal changes.

Sadly, many of these groups are underrepresented in menopause conversations and research. I want to acknowledge that and highlight the importance of broadening the conversation. Everyone navigating menopause regardless of gender identity, ethnicity, or background deserves to feel seen, valued and empowered.

No matter how or when menopause enters your life, you deserve understanding, compassion and support and I hope this book offers just that.

Three Quick Wins

1. Track your symptoms - Start a simple menopause journal. Jot down any changes in mood, sleep, energy, or body. Tracking helps you spot patterns and take control. You can download the balance app created by Dr. Louise Newson for menopause support and symptom tracking. It's available for free worldwide via this link https://www.balance-menopause.com/balance-app/

2. Ditch the Guilt – However menopause shows up for you, it's not a reflection of your strength or health. Give yourself permission to rest and prioritise yourself without guilt.

3. Rewrite Your Menopause Narrative – Shift your mindset. Write down one positive thing about this stage. Maybe it's caring less about what others think, stepping into confidence, or finally putting yourself first.

---

2 BUILDING THE FOUNDATIONS OF FEELING INCREDIBLE THROUGH MENOPAUSE

"You don't have to make drastic changes to see a difference. Small steps, taken consistently, lead to real transformation"

Michelle Obama

Five Things You'll Learn in this Chapter:

- **HRT is a powerful option,** but it's not the only option.
- **HRT can be excellent** for many women, but if it's not suitable for you, lifestyle changes can significantly support your health and well-being.
- **Small steps** create big change.
- **You don't need to overhaul your life.** Simple habits like hydration, movement, and stress management can greatly improve your energy, mood, and sense of control.
- **Building your 'Menopause Health and Beauty Support Kit' is key.** Creating a personalised kit with nutrition, enjoyable movement, stress reduction and sleep strategies is essential for managing symptoms and feeling balanced.

The HRT Conundrum – A Personal Insight

You're in your 40s and one day, something feels... off. Maybe it's a hot flush creeping up out of nowhere, waking up drenched in sweat, or forgetting someone's name. Maybe you feel anxious or overwhelmed for no reason at all. Then, the word menopause starts circling in your head and before you know it, you're plunged into a world of advice, opinions and solutions.

Everywhere you turn, HRT is often the go-to answer, at least in some parts of the world. In countries where menopause is openly discussed, the conversation around HRT has grown stronger in recent years, which is fantastic. There's increasing awareness of how it may support bone health, brain function, heart health and even longevity. But this isn't the case everywhere in the world. In some places, access to HRT is limited, menopause is still a taboo topic and doctors aren't always informed of the full range of options available. And while HRT can be a game-changer for many women, where does that leave those of us who can't take it or simply don't want to?

For health reasons, I'm one of those women who can't take HRT. And let me tell you, there have been moments when that fact has left me feeling fearful, frustrated and completely left out of the conversation. I've read articles linking low oestrogen to dementia and thought, "What now? Am I just going to slowly decline with no way to stop it?" I know I'm not alone in this so many women have told me they feel exactly the same.

But here's what I want you to know: you are not powerless. You don't have to sit back and hope for the best. There are so many things you can do to support your body, your mind and your overall well-being. While HRT replaces hormones, it is not the only way to feel strong, vibrant and in control.

Menopause isn't just about getting through it, it's about thriving. It's about stepping into a new phase of life where you feel good, confident and in control of your health and happiness. And the best part? You get to decide what that looks like for you.

This means focusing on the big picture, nutrition, movement, stress management, skin health, sleep and emotional well-being. All of these play a role in how you feel, look and experience menopause. Every small action you take adds up. Whether it's eating foods that fuel your energy, getting outside for some movement, or simply giving yourself permission to slow down, these daily choices shape how you feel.

This is why I believe every woman should have her own "Menopause toolkit" or, as I like to call it, your Menopause Health and Beauty Support Kit. This isn't about deprivation or unrealistic routines. It's about real, practical strategies that work for you whether that's eating to support your hormones, finding stress relieving techniques that actually help, or discovering ways to sleep better so you wake up feeling like yourself again.

And let's talk about emotions. Hormonal shifts can turn the volume up on anxiety, irritability, or even moments of feeling completely out of sorts. That's normal. Knowing that your feelings are influenced by these changes can help you give yourself patience and understanding. This isn't about 'coping' it's about owning your menopause journey in a way that works for you.

"Menopause isn't about just getting through, it's about reclaiming your health and well-being. Whether you choose HRT or not, the way you care for yourself can create profound changes. With the right tools and mindset, you can feel strong, vibrant and truly yourself again."

So to every woman who can't or doesn't want to take HRT: you are not alone. And let me be clear, I fully support the women who choose to take HRT. It's an incredible tool and for many, it's life-changing. But if it's not for you, that doesn't mean you're out of options.

You have so much more power than you think. The choices you make today, small, simple, doable choices can completely shift how you experience this stage of life. This is your journey. You get to decide what works for you.

There's also an evolving conversation around HRT use for women with a history of hormone-sensitive cancers. While it was once strictly avoided, some emerging research is beginning to explore when and how it might be considered safe in certain cases. This is still a delicate, ongoing area of study, and it's absolutely essential to have a thorough conversation with your healthcare provider about what's right for your unique medical history.

"Menopause is when the universe gently places her hands upon

your shoulders, pulls you close

and whispers in your ear:

'I'm not screwing around. It's time.'"

Adapted from Brené Brown

Small Wins Lead to Big Changes

The good news is you don't have to overhaul your whole life at once to see improvements. Every day, I see how my clients benefit profoundly from small, manageable changes that fit seamlessly into their daily routines. Start small, build momentum and keep it practical. I'm a great believer in keeping things simple!

What we do daily adds up to our overall well-being. Going back to my 80/20 rule, well 90 /10 (10% are pleasure foods) as we come into menopause. It's these daily habits that make all the difference. To sustain a lifestyle that is positive for your health, it's all about taking small steps because small changes are easier to stick to and are more sustainable long-term.

One small change could be adding a handful of leafy greens, like spinach or kale, to one of your meals each day. This can boost your magnesium levels, which helps to ease symptoms such as cramps or mood swings. Starting with things you can achieve and you can do daily builds confidence and seeing results keeps you motivated.

I see so many women trying to change everything at once. Maybe they can sustain it for a few weeks but then they stop because it's just not realistic. This leads to a feeling of having failed and a vicious cycle of guilt can set in.

Client story

Rachel came to me feeling completely defeated. She had tried to change everything at once cutting out all sugar, overhauling her diet and committing to an intense exercise routine 'overnight'. She managed it for a few weeks, but eventually, it all became too much and she ended up giving up, feeling worse than before. The guilt of not being able to keep it up made her feel like she had failed.

When we began working together, I suggested she take a step back and focus on just one change at a time. We started with something simple: adding more water to her day. Once she got comfortable with that, we added in a 10-minute daily walk. Slowly, Rachel started to see positive results and instead of feeling overwhelmed, she began to feel stronger and happier in her daily life. Small, sustainable changes became the building blocks of her success, helping her escape that vicious cycle of guilt, and regain her confidence.

Stories like this remind us that small, intentional changes can have a powerful impact on how we feel every day. You don't have to overhaul your entire life to start noticing improvements. It's the simplest habits that make the biggest difference. Here's a list of easy, actionable steps to help you feel more energised, balanced and in control.

Small Steps, Big Impact:
Easy Changes to Improve How You Feel

Small Change	What does it do?
Drink an extra glass of water	Helps reduce brain fog and improves energy levels
Five-minute morning stretch	Eases muscle tension, boosts circulation and reduces stiffness
Eat a protein-packed breakfast	Stabilises blood sugar, reducing fatigue; helps with weight management and irritability throughout the day
Deep breathing for five minutes	Lowers stress levels, reduces anxiety and helps with mood regulation
Add an extra portion of greens	Supports hormonal balance and improves skin health due to antioxidants
Take a 10-minute walk outside	Boosts endorphins, helps maintain bone density and improves mood

Building Consistency –

How Simple Routines Can Bring Back Control

Menopause can be an unpredictable time in a woman's life. It can make you feel like everything is out of control. That's why establishing routines is such a powerful tool to help you on your way to feeling great again. But what does routine actually mean?

The dictionary definition is "a sequence of actions regularly followed". Routines should be easy to implement and should not feel like a burden. They help bring a sense of control, especially when menopause can make life feel chaotic. Routines can centre around what you do before you go to bed or what you do in the mornings before you start your day. Research shows that having routines particular around exercise, sleep and stress management can help ease menopausal symptoms.

Aim for consistency not perfection

You can start with one simple routine like waking up at the same time each day or deciding not to reach for your phone as soon as you wake up, create a morning routine that sets you up for the day. Here is an example of my morning routine:

- **Hydrate**: Drink a glass of water as soon as you wake up.

- **Stretch**: Do a 5-minute stretch or light yoga to wake your body and get you moving.

- **Skincare**
    - Cleanse your face with a gentle, hydrating cleanser and use a toner.
    - Apply a vitamin C serum followed by a moisturiser with hyaluronic acid.
    - Always finish with SPF 30+ for skin protection.

- **Quick Balanced Breakfast**: Greek yogurt with fresh berries and a handful of nuts.

- **Set an Intention**: Take one minute to set a positive intention for your day.

Routines can also have a positive effect on your emotional well-being. Hormonal fluctuations can mean you experience changes in your moods, leaving you irritated over tiny things or becoming anxious easily. Establishing a regular schedule helps create a sense of stability, which positively impacts your emotional well-being. Routines bring a sense of purpose and a small sense of achievement every day, which can be especially helpful during times when you might feel overwhelmed.

Small routines are powerful tools for navigating menopause. I understand that life doesn't always allow for perfect adherence, but the goal is to keep trying and create a steady rhythm that helps you feel a bit more in control.

Next, you'll discover how nourishing your body with the right foods can help balance your hormones, boost your energy and support you during this transition.

"A routine doesn't have to be grand; it just has to be yours. Every small habit you nurture brings you closer to feeling better and feeling like yourself again."

Start your day by setting one intention, something small, like "I will prioritise myself today" or "I'll take five minutes for myself." This grounding habit can give your morning purpose and help you feel more in control.

Three Quick Wins

1. Don't Look at Your Phone First Thing - Instead of scrolling, take a few deep breaths, stretch, or enjoy a quiet moment to start your day with intention.

2. Make One Simple Swap - Swap a processed snack for nuts or fruit or trade one coffee for herbal tea. Small changes add up.

3. Start a Quick Morning Routine (Even Just 5 Minutes) - Do a simple stretch, drink a glass of water, or step outside for fresh air. A small, consistent morning habit can set a positive tone for the day.

3 NOURISH FOR BALANCE:
EATING FOR HORMONAL HARMONY

"Food isn't just fuel, it's information. Every bite you eat sends instructions to your body, shaping your hormones, energy, mood and how you show up in the world"

Alison Bladh

Five Things You'll Learn in this Chapter:

- **Eat to Support Your Hormones.** The right nutrition can ease the transition through perimenopause and menopause. Simple dietary changes can improve your energy, mood, skin, and overall wellbeing.

- **Focus on Blood Sugar Balance.** Balanced meals that include protein, healthy fats, and fibre help keep your blood sugar steady — reducing energy dips, cravings, irritability, and mood swings.

- **Add in Phytoestrogens.** Foods like flaxseeds, tofu, tempeh, and chickpeas contain plant compounds that mimic oestrogen and may help relieve hot flushes and other hormonal symptoms.

- **Magnesium and Omega-3s are Essential.** These powerful nutrients support brain health, reduce inflammation, and improve sleep all vital during the menopausal transition.

- **Consider a Mediterranean Approach.** A Mediterranean-style diet rich in colourful veg, healthy fats, legumes, and fish can reduce symptoms, protect your heart, and support long-term health.

Hormones influence everything, from mood, energy and metabolism to skin health and sleep. As oestrogen and progesterone begin to shift during perimenopause, many women start noticing changes they never expected. The good news? The way you eat can have a profound impact on how you feel.

While food isn't a magic fix that can replace hormones, it's one of the most powerful tools you have to support your body through this transition. The right nutrition can help stabilise energy, manage symptoms and even improve your mood, skin and overall well-being. But with so much conflicting information out there, it can be overwhelming to know what actually works!

I see the impact of food every day in my work. It's not about dieting or cutting everything out, it's about nourishing your body in a way that helps you feel your best. The choices you make on your plate can either fuel exhaustion or restore vitality, increase inflammation or calm it and support balance or throw things further out of sync.

In this chapter, we'll explore how to nourish your body in a way that supports it, rather than fights against it, helping you feel stronger, happier, more balanced and in control.

The Power of Nutrition During Menopause

Certain nutrients and foods can help naturally support hormonal balance and provide relief from common symptoms like joint pain, weight gain, mood swings and brain fog. For example:

Phytoestrogens are plant compounds that can mimic oestrogen in the body. Foods like flaxseeds (linseeds), soy products and chickpeas are rich in phytoestrogens and may alleviate menopausal symptoms. A meta-analysis by Chedraui et al. (2013) showed that phytoestrogens were linked to a reduction in the frequency of hot flushes. Recent insights from the ZOE study suggest that a daily intake of 15 mg of genistein, an isoflavone found in soy products, may effectively alleviate menopausal symptoms such as hot flushes and night sweats. This dosage aligns with findings from other research, which indicate that genistein can mimic oestrogen in the body, offering relief during perimenopause and menopause. Incorporating genistein-rich foods like soy milk, tofu and edamame into your diet may help achieve this intake, supporting hormonal balance and overall well-being during this transitional phase.

Magnesium supports relaxation, reduces anxiety and promotes better sleep, all of which are common challenges during menopause. Foods like spinach, almonds and pumpkin seeds are excellent sources and a study by Tarleton et al. (2017) highlighted magnesium's role in improving sleep quality.

Omega-3 fatty acids have powerful anti-inflammatory properties and play a crucial role in improving brain health, which becomes especially important as oestrogen levels drop. Found in foods like salmon, flaxseeds, marine algae and chia seeds, omega-3s can help reduce brain fog, enhance concentration and protect your heart and bones. Research by Yurko-Mauro et al. (2010) demonstrated that omega-3 supplementation improved cognitive function, making it particularly valuable during menopause. Unfortunately, many of us are deficient in these essential fatty acids yet they are vital for managing symptoms and supporting overall health. Incorporating omega-3-rich foods into your diet regularly can make a noticeable and positive difference.

A Foundation for Hormonal Harmony

Maintaining stable blood sugar by reducing refined sugars and processed foods is key. Fluctuating oestrogen levels can intensify mood swings and energy dips, but a balanced, nutrient-rich diet can help mitigate these effects and promote steadier energy and mood. If you take just one thing from this book, blood sugar balance should be it! Getting it right can have a huge effect on your overall health during menopause and beyond.

One style of eating consistently stands out in research: the Mediterranean diet. Based on whole foods like vegetables, fish, seafood, whole grains and healthy fats, it's both delicious and sustainable. A study by Llaneza et al. (2012) found that women following a Mediterranean diet reported fewer menopausal symptoms and a better quality of life.

Food as a Supportive Ally

While no single food or supplement can replace your hormones, focusing on supportive nutrition is one of the most powerful tools you have. By working with your body's changing needs, you can stay balanced and in control. Nutrition isn't just about managing symptoms; it's about helping you feel better as you move through this new stage of life.

Understanding Balanced Eating for Hormonal Health: A Step Towards Feeling Better Now

What you eat during menopause can have a profound impact on how you experience symptoms. For instance, studies show that diets high in sugar and ultra-processed carbohydrates worsen symptoms. I know that life can be busy and the question I'm often asked is: "What should I eat?" But before we look into what to eat, let's first talk about how we should eat.

This chapter focuses on balanced eating, what it means and why it matters during menopause. In the next chapter, we'll explore weight management, but for now, let's start with this foundational approach to nourishing your body.

What is Balanced Eating?

Balanced eating means including protein, healthy fats and complex carbohydrates in every meal and snack. As you move into your 40s and beyond, your body begins to change in ways that can feel confusing and overwhelming. Hormones fluctuate, energy dips and you might notice weight redistributing or mood swings happening more often. Amidst all these changes, balanced eating can make a world of difference.

This isn't about rigid rules or the latest diet trend; it's about providing your body with the nutrients it needs to support you during this transition. As oestrogen and progesterone levels fluctuate, your nutritional needs shift too. The way you eat can either help stabilise your hormones and energy or leave you feeling sluggish, irritable and struggling with your weight.

How Balanced Eating Supports You

Incorporating meals with the right balance of protein, healthy fats and wholegrain/complex carbohydrates helps regulate your blood sugar levels, which is not only key for maintaining steady energy throughout the day, but is crucial for managing common menopause symptoms like:

- Hot flushes
- Mood swings
- Sleep disruptions
- Energy slumps
- Anxiety

Here's how each nutrient plays its part:

Protein: Helps you feel full for longer, supports weight management, and is essential for maintaining muscle mass which naturally declines as we age. It also plays a key role in stabilising mood and supporting healthy skin, hair and nails.

Healthy Fats: Found in foods like avocados, nuts, seeds and oily fish, healthy fats support hormone production, brain health and mental clarity, helping you stay sharp and focused.

Wholegrain Carbohydrates: Fibre-rich carbs like oats, quinoa and brown rice provide steady energy, improve digestion and support gut health, all of which is crucial for hormonal balance. Don't forget, vegetables are also a source of carbohydrates and play an important role in providing fibre, vitamins and antioxidants.

"Nourishing your body isn't about kale smoothies every day, it's about enjoying the cake without eating the whole thing (well, most of the time)!"

Why It Matters?

Balanced eating is more than just a healthy habit, it's a tool for reclaiming how you feel. When your body gets the nutrients it needs, you're not only fuelling your day but actively helping to manage the hormonal shifts that come with menopause. This isn't about perfection; it's about making simple, intentional choices that support your health and well-being.

By the end of this chapter, you'll have a clear understanding of how to approach balanced eating and feel more confident in making food choices that work for you during this life phase.

Best Order to Eat Meals to Avoid Blood Sugar Spikes

Eating foods in a strategic order can help stabilise blood sugar levels, reduce energy crashes and support hormonal balance. Follow this simple structure when eating.

Order	What to Eat	Why It Matters	Examples
1. Fibre First	Vegetables, leafy greens, seeds	Slows digestion and prevents rapid blood sugar spikes	Salad, steamed broccoli, flaxseeds
2. Protein Next	Meat, fish, eggs, tofu, legumes	Supports satiety, stabilises energy, and keeps cravings in check	Chicken, salmon, lentils, Greek yogurt
3. Healthy Fats	Avocado, nuts, olive oil, seeds	Slows glucose absorption and supports hormonal balance	Almonds, olive oil, chia seeds
4. Carbs Last	Whole grains, starchy vegetables, fruit	Avoids rapid insulin spikes and helps maintain steady energy	Brown rice, quinoa, sweet potato, berries

---

Tip:

If you're eating a mixed meal (like a salad with wholegrains and protein), start with fibre and protein, then eat your healthy fats and finish with carbs. This simple strategy can improve blood sugar control and prevent energy crashes.

"You wouldn't run a car on the wrong fuel and expect it to work properly. Your body deserves the same care"

Unknown

Fig.3 Balanced Eating Plate

Your Balanced Eating Plate

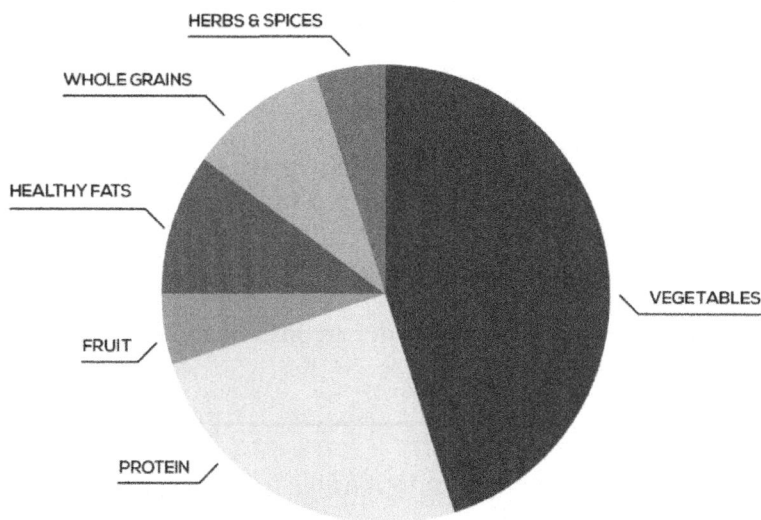

HERBS & SPICES

WHOLE GRAINS

HEALTHY FATS

VEGETABLES

FRUIT

PROTEIN

45% Vegetables
Colourful, fibre-rich veg – cruciferous
types like broccoli, cauliflower and
Brussels sprouts, plus carrots, peppers,
courgette, leafy greens and a little
sauerkraut or kimchi.

10% Healthy Fats
Nuts, olive oil, seeds,
coconut oil, avocados, butter,
full-fat natural yoghurt

25% Protein
Eggs, tempeh, tofu, organic poultry,
oily fish, white fish, legumes, pulses,
quinoa, edamame, seeds, nuts,
full-fat Greek yoghurt

10% Whole Grains
Quinoa, brown rice,
buckwheat, oats

5% Fruit
Low-sugar, whole fruits – berries,
apples, pears, kiwis. Eat a rainbow for
antioxidants and vitamins.

5% Herbs & Spices
Enhance flavour with basil,
parsley, coriander, mint, turmeric,
garlic and ginger.

Everyday Tips for Eating Well in Menopause

- Choose whole, unprocessed foods whenever possible
- Cut back on sugar
- Be mindful with caffeine and alcohol
- Stay hydrated, your body thrives on water!

Healthy eating doesn't have to be boring. A client once told me, 'You are the only person I know that make vegetables sound sexy!' And that's exactly my goal to make nutritious choices irresistible.

The Role of Insulin and Blood Sugar in Menopause

As we've already talked about, menopause is a time of hormonal upheaval, but it's not just your reproductive hormones that are in the spotlight. Two key players to consider are insulin and cortisol.

Insulin: This hormone is responsible for managing your blood sugar levels. During menopause, hormonal changes can lead to insulin resistance, meaning your cells don't respond as well to insulin. This can cause blood sugar spikes and crashes, affecting your energy, mood, weight, and even skin health.

Cortisol: Often referred to as the stress hormone, cortisol levels can increase during menopause. This not only heightens stress and anxiety but also affects blood sugar regulation, leading to cravings, energy dips and a tougher time managing weight. While cortisol's role in menopause is significant, we'll dive deeper into its effects and how to manage stress in Chapter 8.

Understanding how these hormones influence your body during menopause is key to recognising the importance of blood sugar balance, something that affects how you feel every day.

When we eat refined carbohydrates (what I tend to call white foods as they have been stripped of fibre) they are very quickly broken down by our digestive system. This means the glucose (i.e. the sugar levels) in our blood increase quickly causing an insulin response. Insulin allows your body to utilise the glucose and your blood sugar drops back down to a normal to a low level, as insulin is very good at what it does! When your blood sugar crashes, you feel tired, exhausted, irritable and your brain will tell you to get some more energy fast! I can assure you it won't be sending you to the broccoli salad or the lentil soup. It will send you to the biscuit tin or the bowl of sweets someone has on their desk at work.

So, let's say you end up at the biscuit tin and eat a few, maybe with a cup of coffee. This will once again shoot your blood sugar up because you've consumed refined carbs and yes, coffee (or the caffeine in it) also influences blood sugar levels. So your blood sugar is now high again and good old insulin is sent out to deal with it and you guessed it, it crashes again. As you can see this is a pattern that goes on throughout the day.

Fig.4 Blood Sugar Rollercoaster

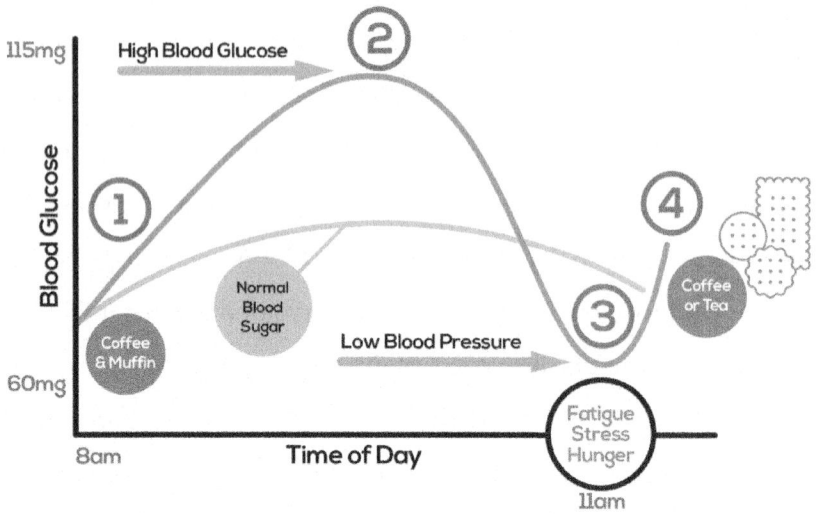

Balanced blood sugar means more than avoiding cravings. It's the key to feeling your best every day.

You may be asking, "Yes, ok, but why does that matter to me?".

The reason it matters, especially during menopause, is this….

Why Blood Sugar Balance Matters During Menopause

During menopause, hormonal changes make your body more prone to blood sugar fluctuations and this can have a significant impact on how you feel daily. Here's why managing your blood sugar is crucial:

Increased insulin resistance

During menopause, lower oestrogen levels can lead to insulin resistance, which means your body has a harder time using glucose effectively. This raises your risk for type 2 diabetes and makes it easier to gain weight, especially around the belly. Insulin resistance can also affect your skin health and contribute to increased signs of ageing.

Mood swings, energy dips and cognitive health

When your blood sugar spikes and crashes, it causes energy dips, irritability and cravings for more sugar. These fluctuations can also worsen symptoms, like brain fog, making it harder to concentrate. Stable blood sugar levels are essential to maintaining steady energy, mood and better cognitive function throughout the day.

Higher Stress and Cortisol Levels

Blood sugar crashes can increase the production of stress hormones like cortisol, which can make anxiety worse and disrupt your sleep. Elevated cortisol also makes it harder to maintain a healthy weight, something many women struggle with during menopause. Cortisol and blood sugar imbalance can also affect hair health, contributing to hair loss and thinning.

Hot Flushes and Night Sweats

High sugar and refined carbohydrates can make hot flushes worse. Balancing blood sugar can help reduce the severity of these symptoms, giving you more control over how often or how intensely they occur.

Weight Gain and Overeating

Spikes and crashes in blood sugar drive cravings, leading to overeating especially sugary foods. This becomes a vicious cycle that makes weight management even harder during menopause. Keeping blood sugar balanced helps curb cravings and supports a healthier relationship with food. We will talk about this more in chapter 4.

Impact on Hair and Skin Health

Blood sugar balance also plays a role in your hair and skin health. Fluctuating blood sugar levels can impact nutrient delivery to hair follicles, potentially contributing to hair thinning. It can also affect the overall health and moisture of your skin, exacerbating common menopausal skin issues like dryness. Eating a high-sugar diet causes what's known as sugar sag! Yes, sugar ages your skin!

To understand the importance of blood sugar balance, let me give you an example of what happens when you start your day with a high sugar breakfast. Let's call this lady Rebecca.

Rebecca is a busy woman, always running short of time in the morning. To get a quick start to her day she often grabs a sugary breakfast cereal or a muffin with her coffee as her go-to breakfast. It seems like a fast and easy way to get some energy, but here's what actually happens in her body.

Starting her day with a high-sugar (as in refined carbohydrates) breakfast causes Rebecca's blood sugar to spike quickly. When sugar enters the bloodstream in large amounts, her body releases insulin which is a hormone that helps move sugar from the blood into her cells, where it's used for energy or stored for later use. During menopause, the body's response to insulin can change, sometimes leading to what's known as insulin resistance. This means her cells become less sensitive to insulin, making it harder for them to use the glucose effectively.

The sugar spike gives her a quick boost of energy, but what goes up must come down. Soon after, Rebecca experiences a blood sugar crash. This leaves her feeling tired, irritable and craving more sugar or caffeine to lift her energy again. This cycle of spikes and crashes not only affects her mood and energy but also adds stress to her body, making her menopause symptoms like fatigue, brain fog and even hot flushes feel more intense.

If Rebecca opted for a balanced breakfast with protein, healthy fats and fibre instead, her blood sugar would rise more gradually. An example of this could be eggs with avocado and wholegrain toast. This steadier blood sugar level helps her feel fuller for longer, keeps her energy stable throughout the morning and makes it easier for her body to manage insulin levels. A balanced breakfast could make all the difference to how Rebecca feels and functions during the day, especially in the midst of perimenopause or menopause.

Practical Blood Sugar Balancing Strategies

So, what can you do to keep your blood sugar balanced? It starts with making intentional food choices that support steady energy levels and minimise those frustrating crashes. Planning your meals in a balanced way doesn't have to be complicated or restrictive.

Below, I've outlined a simple four-day meal plan to inspire you. These are just ideas to show how straightforward it can be to eat in a way that keeps your blood sugar stable while still enjoying delicious, nourishing food. The goal here isn't to follow this exactly but to give you a framework to build upon.

Everyone's body is different and how we respond to certain foods can vary widely. Use this plan as a starting point to observe how you feel after meals, experiment with combinations that work for you and make adjustments based on your preferences and what feels good for you.

Did You Know?

Flaxseeds need to be ground for your body to absorb their nutrients. Whole flaxseeds often pass through undigested!
Grind for best absorption - soaking helps but isn't enough.
Ground flaxseeds start to oxidise quickly, so store them in the fridge and use within 3-7 days.
Sprinkle on yogurt, oats, or salads for an easy nutrition boost!

Blood sugar balancing four-day easy meal ideas

Day One

Breakfast: Greek yoghurt topped with mixed berries, a handful of almonds and a sprinkle of chia seeds. (Plant-based: use coconut yoghurt)

Lunch: Wrap-less veggie roll with hummus, cucumber, shredded carrot and avocado rolled in large lettuce leaves.

Dinner: Roasted salmon (or chickpeas for plant-based), sweet potatoes and broccoli on a baking tray season and bake everything together.

Snack: Apple slices with a spoonful of almond butter.

Day Two

Breakfast: Overnight oats with almond milk, chia seeds, sunflower seeds, flaxseeds, nuts of your choice and sliced strawberries.

Lunch: Quinoa mixed with a tin of tuna (or chickpeas for plant-based), cherry tomatoes, diced cucumber and a drizzle of olive oil.

Dinner: Stir-fry with tofu (or chicken), bell peppers, broccoli and sugar snap peas, served with cooked brown rice.

Snack: Handful of mixed nuts and a banana.

Day Three

Breakfast: Scrambled eggs (or tofu) with baby spinach and a sprinkle of pumpkin seeds.

Lunch: Homemade lentil and vegetable soup with a side of cucumber sticks.

Dinner: Baked chicken breast (or tempeh) with steamed vegetables (broccoli, carrots) and quinoa.

Snack: Greek yoghurt with a sprinkle of ground flaxseeds and pumpkin seeds. (Plant-based: use coconut yoghurt).

Day Four

Breakfast: Smoothie with spinach, banana, almond milk, chia seeds, flaxseeds, MCT oil and a scoop of protein powder.

Lunch: Salad with mixed greens, black beans, avocado, diced bell pepper and cooked quinoa and an olive oil dressing.

Dinner: Baked cod (or veggie burger made from beans) with roasted carrots, zucchini and cauliflower on a baking tray.

Snack: Cucumber slices with homemade hummus.

You can also visit my recipe page for inspiration: www.alisonbladh.com/recipes

A Word on Continuous Glucose Monitors (CGMs)

Continuous Glucose Monitors (CGMs) are wearable devices that track your blood sugar in real time using a small sensor on your skin. They can help you understand how meals, snacks, exercise and stress affect your glucose levels, offering personalised insights into your body's unique responses. I have tried one and it was an eye opener! It really made me realise how individual we are in how we react to different foods. Pasta (white) is certainly not something I eat often after seeing how it raised my blood sugar.

For menopausal women, CGMs can be especially helpful in identifying trigger foods, managing energy crashes and fine-tuning meal timing. For example, you might discover that certain "healthy" foods cause unexpected blood sugar spikes or find the ideal balance of nutrients to keep your energy steady.

While CGMs are an excellent tool for understanding patterns, they're not essential for everyone. They can be costly and may require a prescription, depending on your region. However, if you're curious and want tailored insights, they can be a valuable addition to your health journey.

Remember, whether you use a CGM or not, the strategies in this book will guide you in managing blood sugar effectively and feeling your best every day.

Why I love MCT oil

MCT oil, (short for medium-chain triglycerides), is a fantastic addition to your diet whenever you need a quick and reliable energy boost. Derived from coconuts, it's made up of fats that are easily absorbed and converted into energy by your body, no complicated digestion required. I love recommending MCT oil to women because it's not only great for keeping energy levels steady but also supports brain health and focus. It's a simple way to add a little extra nourishment to your day. I love adding it to my matcha tea, but it's equally brilliant drizzled over salads or blended into your morning coffee or porridge for an effortless health upgrade.

When buying MCT oil, look for a high-quality, pure product made from 100% coconut oil, avoiding blends with palm oil or unnecessary additives.

Food Choices: What to Enjoy and What to Limit

Let's be realistic: food is one of life's greatest pleasures. We all love food! It's not just fuel; it's social, comforting and meant to be enjoyed. That's why balance is the key, not deprivation. I'm a big believer in keeping things simple and practical, so let's talk about the 90/10 rule again: focus on nourishing your body with good choices 90% of the time, leaving room for those occasional indulgences (what I call pleasure foods) that make life sweeter without guilt or regret.

Below, you'll find two lists: foods to prioritise and foods to limit for better blood sugar balance and overall wellness during menopause. This isn't about cutting things out completely; it's about making intentional choices that help you feel your best. It's all about balance and yes, you can still enjoy your favourite treats while keeping your health in mind.

Take Action!

I want you to go into your kitchen and get a big bin bag and throw away all the junk food, all the ultra-processed foods what I call the 'white stuff'. Have a clear out because it's a great place to start. Now you've taken away the temptation of all those trigger foods that are not nourishing your body, you can replace them with all the nourishing foods that will make you feel great. Next, you can go food shopping but don't buy any of the junk. Focus on stocking your kitchen with wholesome, nutrient-rich foods that will energise you and support your health.

I've created a downloadable list for you so you can print it off and have it on your fridge as a reminder.

Nourishing food choices for Menopause:
What to Enjoy and What to Limit or Avoid

Foods to Enjoy		
Food	**Why**	**Sources**
Leafy Greens	Rich in magnesium, calcium, and antioxidants which help manage stress, support bone health, and reduce inflammation.	Spinach, kale, Swiss chard, collard greens
Cruciferous Vegetables	Support hormone balance and liver detoxification.	Broccoli, Brussels sprouts, cauliflower, cabbage
Berries	High in antioxidants that benefit brain health, reduce inflammation, and support skin elasticity	Blueberries, raspberries, strawberries, blackberries
Whole Grains	Provide complex carbohydrates to stabilise blood sugar, support energy levels, and aid digestion	Oats, quinoa, brown rice, barley
Healthy Fats	Support hormone production, heart	Avocado, olive oil, flaxseed oil,

	health, joint health, and skin hydration	coconut oil, butter, nuts and seeds
Fatty Fish	High in omega-3s, which support brain function, reduce inflammation, and protect the heart	Salmon, mackerel, sardines, trout
Nuts and Seeds	Provide protein, fibre, healthy fats and phytoestrogens, which may help ease symptoms	Flaxseeds, chia seeds, almonds, walnuts
High-Quality Protein	Helps maintain muscle mass, stabilises blood sugar, and supports energy and mood	Lean meats, eggs, Greek yogurt, chickpeas, lentils
Phytoestrogen-Rich Foods	Contain plant-based compounds that may help ease symptoms like hot flushes and mood swings	Flaxseeds, soybeans, tofu, tempeh
Legumes	Rich in fibre and phytoestrogens, helping to balance blood sugar and support hormone health	Chickpeas, black beans, lentils, edamame

Fermented Foods	Improve gut health, which supports digestion, immune function and mood	Yogurt, kefir, kimchi, sauerkraut
Bone-Building Foods	Supply calcium and vitamin D to maintain bone density during and after menopause	Sardines (with bones), fortified almond milk, tofu, collard greens
Herbal Teas and Infusions	Provide antioxidants, support hydration, aid sleep and soothe digestion	Green tea, chamomile, lemon balm, peppermint, rooibos
Sea Vegetables	Rich in iodine and trace minerals that support thyroid function and hormone metabolism	Nori, wakame, dulse (dried flakes or sheets added to meals)
Pumpkin Seeds	High in magnesium, zinc, and tryptophan — great for mood, sleep, and hormonal balance	Add to salads, porridge, or smoothies
Eggs	Provide high-quality protein, healthy fats, and choline for brain and liver health, plus skin and hair support	Boiled, poached, scrambled, or in frittatas
Dark Chocolate (min. 70%)	A natural mood booster, rich in	A few small squares as a

	magnesium and antioxidants. Can help reduce stress and manage cravings	mindful treat
Mushrooms	Support immune health and liver detoxification. Some (like reishi) may help regulate oestrogen	Shiitake, maitake, reishi and lion's mane add to stir-fries, soups, or teas
Beetroot	Supports liver detox, circulation, and energy levels	Roasted, grated raw, or juiced
Turmeric	Powerful anti-inflammatory spice that may help ease joint pain, support liver health, and improve mood	Add to stews, soups, or as golden milk with black pepper

Foods to Limit or Avoid

Food	Why	Sources
Ultra-Processed Foods	High in sugars, unhealthy fats, additives and preservatives that can promote inflammation, blood sugar imbalances, fatigue, and weight gain.	Ready meals, packaged snacks, sugary cereals, sweets
Sugary Snacks and Drinks	Spike blood sugar and insulin levels, leading to energy crashes, mood swings, brain fog and increased hot flushes	Sweets, fizzy drinks, pastries, flavoured yoghurts
Refined Carbohydrates	Rapidly digested carbs can worsen cravings, mood changes, weight gain and hormone disruption	White bread, white pasta, white rice, rice cakes, cakes, biscuits
Caffeine	Can overstimulate the nervous system, disrupt sleep and worsen anxiety or hot flushes, especially later in the day	Coffee, black tea, green tea, energy drinks, cola
Processed Meats	High in sodium,	Sausages, bacon,

	saturated fats, and preservatives, which may increase inflammation, blood pressure and cancer risk	ham, salami, deli meats
High-Sodium Foods	Can cause water retention, bloating, increased hot flushes, and raise blood pressure over time	Salmon, mackerel, sardines, trout
Spicy Foods	Can act as a trigger for hot flushes and night sweats in some women, worsening discomfort	Hot sauces, curries, spicy takeaways, chilli-based seasonings
Fried Foods and Trans Fats	Promote inflammation, increase bad cholesterol, and contribute to heart risk and weight gain	Fried chicken, chips, doughnuts, deep-fried snacks, processed baked goods
Artificial Sweeteners	May cause bloating, affect gut health, and worsen cravings and insulin sensitivity in some women	Aspartame, sucralose, saccharin, found in diet drinks and sugar-free foods
Excessive Red Meat	Can increase inflammation and oxidative stress when	Large portions of beef, lamb, pork. **Tip:** Choose

	eaten in large amounts, affecting hormone balance	organic or wild meat and enjoy in moderation
Low-Fibre Foods	Lacking in fibre, these foods can slow digestion, affect gut health and worsen bloating and fatigue	White crackers, white bread, processed breakfast cereals, white carbohydrates
Flavoured Yogurts	Often high in added sugars and artificial flavourings, which can spike blood sugar and affect mood or energy	Fruit yoghurts, dessert-style yoghurts, low-fat flavoured pots
Energy Drinks and Fruit Juice	High in sugar, caffeine or stimulants, which may disrupt sleep, raise stress hormones and worsen symptoms	Energy drinks, pre-workout drinks or fruit juice

Meal Timing for Menopause and Hormone Balance

There's been a lot of buzz around intermittent fasting in recent years. You've probably seen it on social media or heard about it in conversation. Maybe you've wondered if it's for you, or perhaps you've already given it a try. In my practice, I've seen some fantastic results with clients who use this approach, particularly during menopause, where it can offer significant benefits.

At its core, intermittent fasting is about eating within a specific time window and giving your body a longer break from food. Research shows that this simple change can do wonders for blood sugar balance, weight management, energy levels, skin health and inflammation reduction. Dr Mindy Pelz, author of Fast Like a Girl, highlights how fasting can also activate autophagy a natural process where your body clears out damaged cells, helping you regenerate and repair. It's a bit like it gives your body a chance to take out the rubbish. This is particularly exciting during menopause, as it offers another layer of support for overall wellness, from reducing inflammation to promoting healthier skin and cellular renewal.

How can Fasting Support Hormonal Health during Menopause?

Intermittent fasting doesn't just help with weight and energy; it also positively influences hormone balance. Studies suggest it can improve insulin sensitivity and regulate leptin, the hormone that signals fullness, which can help with appetite control and metabolism regulation.

Fasting also gives your digestive system a break, which may reduce bloating and improve overall gut health, a common concern during menopause. By allowing time for rest and repair, it supports your microbiome, giving those all-important good gut bugs a chance to thrive. This connection between gut health and hormone balance is essential, as the gut plays a significant role in metabolising hormones and supporting overall health during menopause.

Dr. Mindy Pelz also explains how intermittent fasting can align with your natural hormonal rhythms. For menopausal women, fasting can stabilise insulin and cortisol levels, helping you feel more balanced and in control. Shorter fasting windows, like 12 to 14 hours, may work better if you're just starting or feeling stressed, while longer fasting windows (up to 16 hours) can enhance fat burning and metabolic benefits when your body is ready.

The Role of Autophagy in Menopause

One of the most exciting benefits of intermittent fasting is its ability to activate autophagy, your body's natural "cell-cleaning" process. During fasting, your body clears out damaged cells and recycles cellular components, paving the way for regeneration and repair. This process is particularly relevant during menopause, as it can help reduce oxidative stress, support skin health and protect brain function.

Autophagy is also linked to reducing systemic inflammation, a key factor in managing menopausal symptoms and maintaining overall health.

"The key to lasting health isn't just what you eat, but how and when you eat."

Dr. Sara Gottfried,

(Hormone and longevity expert)

Skin and Longevity Benefits of Fasting

Emerging research suggests intermittent fasting may improve skin hydration, texture, and overall appearance by reducing systemic inflammation, which can exacerbate conditions like acne and psoriasis. Additionally, autophagy supports skin regeneration, helping maintain a more youthful glow, a welcome bonus during menopause, when hormonal changes can affect skin elasticity and moisture. Beyond skin, fasting's anti-inflammatory effects may lower the risks of chronic conditions like heart disease and diabetes, which are increasingly important to manage as we age.

Examples of Fasting Windows

Example of a 10-Hour Fasting Window:
Start: 8.00pm
Finish: 6.00am

Time	Meal	Food
6.00am	Balanced Breakfast	Scrambled eggs with smoked salmon and avocado on a slice of wholegrain toast. (Vegan alternative: Scrambled tofu with turmeric, nutritional yeast, and avocado on wholegrain toast.)
12.30pm	Nourishing Lunch	Grilled chicken or grilled tempeh with roasted butternut squash, steamed asparagus, and a quinoa salad with olive oil dressing.

| 4.30pm | Light Snack | A small handful of almonds, a few squares of dark chocolate, or hummus with sliced cucumber and carrot sticks. |
| 7.00pm | Dinner | Baked salmon with roasted Brussels sprouts and mashed cauliflower. (Vegan alternative: Baked tofu or chickpea patties with the same sides.) |

This 10-hour fasting window provides enough time for the body to digest and recover overnight while ensuring balanced energy, blood sugar control, and hormone support throughout the day.

Example of a 12-Hour Fasting Window:
Start: 7.00pm
Finish: 7.00am

Time	Meal	Food
7.00am	Balanced Breakfast	Chia pudding made with unsweetened almond milk, topped with berries and a sprinkle of flaxseeds.
12.00pm	Nourishing Lunch	Grilled turkey or marinated tempeh with quinoa, roasted bell peppers, and a salad of leafy greens.
4.00pm	Light Snack	A small handful of pumpkin seeds, Greek yoghurt or coconut yoghurt

		with a sprinkle of cinnamon, or cucumber slices with guacamole.
6.00pm	Dinner	A hearty vegetable soup with lentils or chickpeas and a slice of wholegrain bread. (Vegan alternative: Same, as it's already plant-based.)

This 12-hour eating window provides a more accessible starting point while offering benefits for metabolic health and digestion.

Example of a 16-Hour Fasting Window:
Start: 6.00pm
Finish: 10.00am

Time	Meal	Food
10.00am	Balanced Breakfast	Scrambled eggs or scrambled tofu with sautéed spinach and cherry tomatoes, served with a slice of whole-grain toast and a drizzle of olive oil. (Vegan alternative: Scrambled tofu with nutritional yeast for a savoury flavour.)
1.30pm	Nourishing Lunch	Grilled chicken or tofu with roasted sweet potato, steamed broccoli, and a drizzle of olive oil.
4.30pm	Light Snack	A small handful of walnuts, a piece of dark chocolate, or a few slices of

		avocado.
5.30pm	Dinner	Baked cod or grilled tempeh with a side of zucchini noodles (courgetti) tossed in garlic and olive oil.

This 16-hour fasting window gives your body a longer rest period to support digestion, metabolic health and hormone balance.

Tips for Success

Keep It Simple: Start with a 10-12 hour fasting window, which is manageable and lets you sleep through most of it.

Listen to Your Body: If fasting leaves you tired, irritable, or unwell, adjust or stop. It's not for everyone.

Stay Hydrated: Drink water and herbal teas during fasting periods to support energy and digestion. Avoid anything that might set your digestion off, such as coffee with milk or cream, artificial sweeteners, carbonated drinks, or fruit juices. Even seemingly harmless additions, like a splash of milk in tea or a flavoured electrolyte drink, can stimulate digestion and break your fast.

Focus on Quality Meals: Prioritise balanced meals with protein, healthy fats, and fibre to stabilise blood sugar.

Experiment and Adapt: Try different fasting windows and adjust based on what feels right for you.

"Eat less, live longer."

Benjamin Franklin

Who Should Be Cautious with Fasting?

While intermittent fasting can offer incredible benefits, it's not suitable for everyone. If you have a history of eating disorders, are underweight, or have medical conditions like diabetes or hypoglycaemia, fasting might not be the right choice. Pregnant or breastfeeding women should also avoid fasting, as their nutritional needs are different. Always consult your healthcare provider before starting a fasting routine, especially if you're on medication or have specific health concerns.

Remember: it's about what works for you.

Intermittent fasting can be a powerful tool, but it's not the only path to wellness. If it works for you, embrace it. If not, let it go without guilt. The goal is to find a routine that aligns with your unique needs and supports your journey through menopause.

By experimenting and adapting, you can discover if fasting enhances your energy, helps you feel more balanced and fits into your life. Ultimately, this is about finding what works for you so you can thrive through this transformative phase.

We have now explored how nourishing your body with delicious whole foods in balance sets the foundations for everything from our energy levels to how we feel emotionally and even our skin health! Yet as many of us know perimenopause and menopause brings with it some unique challenges, weight management being one of them which can be very frustrating to say the least. This book is not about crash diets and deprivation, it's about understanding your body as it changes and finding solutions that work for you. In the next chapter we will be looking at easy, realistic strategies to help support a healthy weight through this transition without sacrificing your happiness and enjoyment for life.

Ready for More Delicious Ideas?

Eating for hormonal balance doesn't have to be complicated, small, consistent choices make a big difference. If you're looking for simple, nourishing meals that support your energy, mood, skin, and weight, I've created a collection just for you.

You'll find easy, menopause-friendly meals that taste as good as they make you feel. Visit my recipe page for inspiration: www.alisonbladh.com/recipes

Download Your Free 7-Day Menopause Reset Meal Plan

Want a simple way to get started with hormone-friendly eating? Scan the QR code to download my free 7-Day Menopause Reset Meal Plan – packed with easy, delicious recipes designed to boost energy, balance blood sugar, and support your body through menopause.

Or visit: www.alisonbladh.com/7-day-menopause-reset-meal-plan

Supplements to Consider for Nutritional Balance

- **Magnesium** (Glycinate or Citrate) – Supports energy, blood sugar balance, and stress resilience.

- **Vitamin D3 with K2** – Essential for hormone production, immunity and calcium absorption.

- **Omega-3 (EPA & DHA)** – Reduces inflammation and supports hormone, heart, and brain health. Vegans can choose algae-based omega-3.

- **Vitamin B Complex (Activated)** – Aids energy, mood, and oestrogen detoxification.

- **Protein Powder** – Useful if you're not getting enough protein from food; supports metabolism, muscle maintenance and satiety.

- **High-quality multivitamin** – A well-formulated multivitamin can offer broad nutritional support.

Three Quick Wins

1. Add One Extra Plant Food - Toss in a handful of spinach, add chickpeas to your soup, or sprinkle ground flaxseeds on your breakfast. More plants = more fibre, nutrients and hormone-friendly goodness.

2. Try an Earlier Dinner - Aim to finish eating by 7 p.m. and let your body rest overnight. A gentle overnight break can help digestion, reduce bloating and improve energy.

3. Eat Without Distractions -
Put away your phone, sit down and enjoy your food mindfully. Even one calm meal a day supports digestion and helps you feel more satisfied.

4 MASTERING MENOPAUSE WEIGHT GAIN – SIMPLE STRATEGIES THAT WORK

"Weight gain isn't inevitable in menopause. What we eat, how we move and how we care for ourselves makes all the difference."

Dr. Mary Claire Haver

Five Things You'll Learn in this Chapter:

- **Weight Gain Isn't Inevitable.** Menopause makes weight management trickier, but small, consistent changes can help you stay in control and feel confident in your body.

- **Focus on Belly Fat for Health.** Visceral fat around the middle isn't just about appearance, it increases your risk for heart disease, diabetes and inflammation.

- **Nutrition Matters More Than Exercise.** What you eat plays a bigger role in weight loss than how much you move. Focus on real, nutrient-dense foods to support hormone balance.

- **GLP-1 and Weight Management.** GLP-1 medications are gaining attention, but they're not magic fixes. Lifestyle changes still matter most for sustainable results.

- **Supportive Treatments Can Help.** Therapies like lymphatic drainage, dry brushing and cryolipolysis can boost results, especially when combined with healthy habits.

Why Menopause can make Weight Management Tricky

One question I hear daily in my practice is, "Why do I put weight on as I age?" It often creeps on gradually, even when you haven't changed the way you eat or exercise. Maybe you've gone up a clothes size or find your jeans harder to button. Perhaps you just don't feel comfortable in your body anymore. Or maybe you've noticed your shape shifting. You feel your body shape has changed from a pear to an apple!

It's easy to get seduced into wanting to look like we did in our 20s or striving to get back to the weight we were back then. But the truth is, we're not 20 anymore and that's perfectly okay. I'm not saying you don't need to manage your weight as it's really important for your health and well-being. However, it's not about chasing an unrealistic ideal or trying to turn back the clock. It's about feeling good, staying energetic and caring for your amazing body. Managing your weight at this stage of life is about being strong, healthy and gently confident. It's not about being the smallest version of yourself.

Let's shift the focus to realistic, achievable goals that celebrate where you are now. By making sustainable, supportive choices, you can feel your best and embrace this stage of life with vibrancy and strength. Weight gain during menopause is a complex issue and unfortunately, there isn't just one answer. It's multifactorial, influenced by many different factors happening in your body at once.

Let's get one thing clear from the beginning: weight gain in perimenopause and menopause is not inevitable! Hormonal changes can make managing weight more difficult, but maintaining consistent healthy nutritional and lifestyle habits can assist in effective weight management. Yes, it does take some effort and perhaps a few changes, but remember, I'm all about easy implementation. I have seen many of the women I work with successfully lose weight and keep the weight off. It just takes a little bit of determination, motivation and a few changes.

It's not about restriction; it's about choosing foods that nourish your body and help it thrive. It's also about recognising and saying no to foods that lack nutrients and don't nourish your body, negatively impacting your health and waistline.

Did you know?

Did you know nearly 60% of women face unexpected weight gain during menopause, even without changes to their diet or exercise? But here's the good news: gaining weight isn't a foregone conclusion. You can take back control with small, manageable steps that fit into your daily life.

Fig.5 Apple and Pear shape

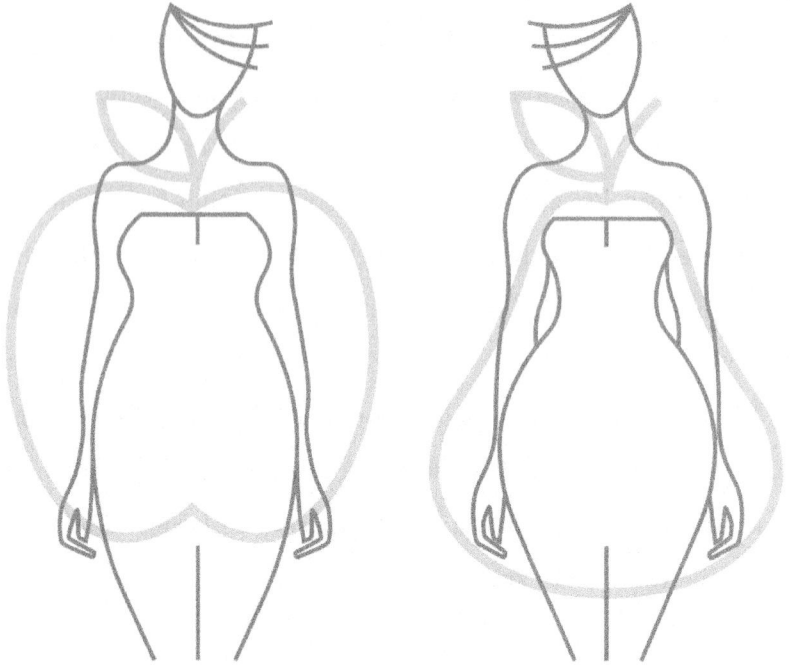

"Declining oestrogen levels during menopause are closely linked to increased fat storage, particularly around the abdomen, highlighting the complex relationship between hormones and body weight"

Why Women Gain Weight during Menopause

If you've noticed the number on the scale creeping up, you're not alone. Many women find that despite eating the same foods and moving just as much (or even more), weight gain still happens. So, what's actually going on?

While researchers are still uncovering all the reasons behind menopausal weight gain, what we do know is that a mix of hormonal changes, lifestyle factors and ageing all play a role. And because every woman's experience is unique, some of these factors may affect you more than others.

Below, you'll find some of the key reasons why managing weight can feel more challenging during this phase of life. But remember, understanding what's happening is the first step because once you know what's driving the change, you can take action to support your body in a way that works for you.

Reasons We Gain Weight

Hormonal Shifts	As oestrogen declines, the body stores more fat, especially around the abdomen, to compensate. Fat tissue produces a weaker form of oestrogen (oestrone), but it's also more inflammatory, contributing to weight gain and metabolic changes.
Slowed Metabolism	Ageing naturally slows

	metabolism, meaning you burn fewer calories at rest. Without adjustments to diet or activity, weight gain becomes easier.
Loss of Muscle Mass	Muscle burns more calories than fat, but declining oestrogen and testosterone levels lead to muscle loss, slowing metabolism further.
Insulin Resistance	Lower oestrogen can make the body less efficient at processing carbs, leading to blood sugar spikes, increased fat storage and energy dips that trigger cravings.
Increased Cortisol from Stress	Higher cortisol levels fuel cravings for sugary, high-fat foods, encourage fat storage around the midsection and break down muscle, further slowing metabolism.
Sleep Disruptions	Poor sleep increases ghrelin (the hunger hormone) and lowers leptin (the fullness hormone), making cravings and overeating more likely. Sleep deprivation also raises cortisol, adding to weight struggles.
Changes in Activity Levels	As we get older, it's common for

	our activity levels to naturally decline. Whether it's due to increased fatigue, joint stiffness, or simply feeling less motivated, many women find themselves moving less than they used to. This drop in daily movement can quietly contribute to weight gain, especially when combined with the hormonal shifts of menopause.
Appetite Changes	Oestrogen is a natural appetite suppressant. As it declines, many women report feeling constantly hungry, never quite satisfied and craving high-calorie comfort foods.
Emotional Eating	Mood swings, anxiety and stress can lead to emotional eating, where food becomes a source of comfort rather than nourishment.
Digestive Changes	Hormonal shifts can slow digestion, leading to bloating, flatulence, constipation and discomfort. A sluggish gut microbiome can also affect

	metabolism and weight.
Thyroid Problems	An underactive thyroid (hypothyroidism) becomes more common with age, slowing metabolism and making weight loss more difficult, even with the right habits.
Medications	Certain medications, including antidepressants, corticosteroids and some blood pressure or diabetes treatments, can contribute to weight gain by increasing appetite, altering metabolism, or promoting fluid retention.
Water Retention	Fluctuating hormones can cause fluid retention, making you feel bloated and heavier, even if you haven't gained actual body fat.
Decreased Growth Hormone Levels	As we age, growth hormone declines, reducing muscle mass and increasing fat accumulation, particularly around the midsection.
Gut Microbiome Changes	Hormonal shifts impact gut bacteria, which play a role in metabolism, digestion, and even

	appetite regulation. A less diverse microbiome may contribute to weight gain.
Less Efficient Nutrient Absorption	Ageing reduces the absorption of key nutrients like protein, B vitamins and magnesium, which can slow metabolism and impact energy levels.
Reduced Brown Fat Activity	Brown fat, also known as brown adipose tissue (BAT), is a type of fat that burns calories to generate heat and help regulate body temperature. Unlike regular white fat, which stores energy, brown fat is metabolically active and helps burn excess calories. However, its activity declines with age, making weight maintenance harder.
More Time Spent Sitting	A busy lifestyle often means more time sitting, whether at work, driving, or relaxing. This slows metabolism and reduces fat-burning efficiency.
Altered Taste Preferences	Hormonal changes can shift taste preferences, increasing cravings for sweet or salty foods without

	you realising it.
Decreased Dopamine Levels	Lower oestrogen reduces dopamine, the "feel-good" hormone, leading to cravings for sugary, processed foods that give a quick mood boost.
Slower Lymphatic System	A sluggish lymphatic system can contribute to bloating, fluid retention and a slower metabolism.
Weakened Detox Pathways	A less efficient liver can slow fat metabolism and increase toxin buildup, affecting energy levels and weight management.
Unconscious Eating & Portion size increase	Portion sizes can unconsciously increase over time. With a slower metabolism, the same amount of food that once maintained weight may now contribute to gradual gain.

Understanding the Health Risks of Menopausal Belly Fat

When it comes to weight loss, it's easy to get caught up in how we look, especially with the changes that often come with menopause. But there's more at stake than fitting into your favourite jeans. During menopause, many women notice an increase in abdominal fat, that stubborn 'menopause belly.' It's important to understand this isn't just an aesthetic issue; it can signal deeper health concerns, specifically related to visceral fat.

What is Visceral Fat?

Visceral fat is the fat that lies deep within the abdomen, surrounding vital organs like the liver, pancreas and intestines. It's different from subcutaneous fat (the fat that sits just under the skin) and is much more dangerous to your health. Visceral fat is more metabolically active, meaning it releases fatty acids and inflammatory markers into the bloodstream, which can raise the risk of serious health conditions.

Why is Visceral Fat Dangerous?

Unlike the fat we can pinch under our skin, visceral fat can have a significant impact on our overall health. Here are some of the main reasons why visceral fat can be harmful:

Heart Health: Increased visceral fat is linked to a higher risk of cardiovascular diseases, including heart attacks and strokes. This is particularly relevant for women post-menopause, as the protective effects of oestrogen decline, raising the risk of heart disease.

Insulin Resistance: Visceral fat contributes to insulin resistance, which can lead to type 2 diabetes. Many women find their blood sugar levels become harder to manage after the age of 40 and this type of fat plays a significant role in that process.

Inflammation: Visceral fat promotes inflammation in the body, increasing the risk of chronic conditions such as arthritis, metabolic syndrome and even certain cancers, including breast cancer.

Why Does Menopause Affect Fat Distribution?

Hormonal changes during perimenopause and menopause play a major role in where fat is stored. As oestrogen levels drop, fat distribution shifts from the hips and thighs to the abdomen. This is partly because oestrogen helps regulate fat distribution and when levels decline, the body compensates by storing fat in the belly. As I said earlier we go from a pear shape to an apple.

On top of that, our metabolism naturally slows as we age and lifestyle factors such as stress, poor sleep and lack of physical activity can exacerbate fat gain in the abdominal area. This is why so many women find it harder to lose weight as they approach menopause.

Focus on Health, Not Just Weight

The good news is that you can manage and reduce visceral fat by making specific lifestyle changes. It's about more than just cutting calories; it's about building long-term habits that support your overall health.

Eat Nutrient-Dense Foods: Prioritise whole foods that help stabilise your blood sugar, like quality protein, healthy fats and fibre-rich vegetables. These not only support steady energy and hormone balance but also help reduce insulin resistance and manage appetite especially when hormonal changes can trigger cravings.

Stay Active: Regular exercise, particularly strength training and aerobic activities, can help reduce visceral fat. Even a brisk daily walk can make a big difference in your long-term health.

Manage Stress: High stress levels contribute to fat storage, especially in the belly, because of the hormone cortisol. Practising relaxation techniques like yoga, meditation, or simply taking time out for yourself can help. The stress hormone cortisol is a fat storing hormone!

Get Enough Sleep: Poor sleep is linked to weight gain and higher levels of visceral fat. Aim for 7-8 hours of good quality sleep each night to support both your metabolism and your overall well-being.

Even though there are challenges, it is possible to maintain your weight or lose weight if that's your goal. I see incredible results with my clients all the time in my practice. It's not about drastic measures; it's about making small, meaningful changes that you can stick with. Sometimes it means doing a U-turn and taking a fresh approach to what you eat, focusing on building habits that are sustainable, enjoyable and work for your lifestyle.

As I've said before, this isn't about restriction or deprivation. It's about finding balance and making choices that support your health in a way that feels good. The key is to take that first step.

Take Action

Set a date for when you're going to start, write it down below and commit to it. Putting a plan in place makes all the difference. Without a clear start, it's easy to keep putting it off, so make that commitment to yourself today. Small, consistent efforts add up to big changes. You have the power to make it happen.

My take action promise:

I, _____, am committing to start my weight management journey on: _____

My first actionable step will be:

_____

Why reaching my weight management goals matters to me:

_____

My promise to myself:

I will take small, consistent steps to prioritise my health and well-being because I deserve to feel strong, confident and in control of my body.

Signed: _____

So, What Can You Do? Sustainable Eating and Lifestyle Habits for Weight Management

So, what can you do? Let's face it, weight management can feel like a challenge during menopause with all the changes happening in your body, but it's absolutely achievable. The key is to focus on sustainable habits that fit into your lifestyle rather than chasing quick fixes that don't last.

Nutrition is one of the most powerful tools you have to support a healthy weight. What we eat, how we eat and even when we eat all make a difference. It's about creating balance and nourishing your body in a way that feels good and is realistic for the long term. If you've actioned what we spoke about in Chapter 3 and cleaned out your cupboards of junk foods that don't serve you, you've already taken a great first step towards making better choices.

Weight Loss Starts in the Kitchen. When it comes to losing weight, what you eat matters more than how much you exercise. In fact, experts often say that weight loss is around 80% nutrition and 20% exercise. That means the food choices you make day-to-day have the biggest impact and that's actually good news, because it puts you in control. You can't out-train a poor diet, but you can nourish your body in a way that supports steady, healthy weight loss.

I know it can be overwhelming to know where to start, especially when life is already busy, but small, manageable changes really do add up. Let's take a closer look at nutrition and the simple things you can do to lose weight and keep it off in a way that works for you.

Realistic Nutrition Changes for Weight Loss in Menopause		
What?	**Why?**	**How?**
Prioritise Protein at Every Meal	Protein helps to preserve muscle mass, which is essential as muscle burns more calories than fat.	Action Step: Include a palm-sized portion of protein such as chicken, fish, eggs, or plant-based options like lentils and tofu in every meal.
Eat More Fibre	Fibre helps regulate digestion, keeps you full longer, detoxifies excess oestrogen, aids elimination, which is really important, and balances blood sugar levels.	Action Step: Add more low sugar fruits, vegetables and whole grains to your diet, aiming for at least 25-30 grams of fibre daily. Snack on high-fibre foods like berries, raw vegetables, sunflower seeds, or nuts.
Choose Healthy Fats	Fats like those in olive oil, avocados and nuts support hormone production and reduce inflammation.	Action Step: Use olive oil for cooking, snack on a handful of almonds, or add avocado to salads.
Balance Carbohydrates	Get rid of the white and go for the brown. Focus on complex	Action Step: Swap refined carbs like white bread for whole grains, such as

	carbohydrates that release energy slowly, preventing blood sugar spikes.	quinoa, brown rice, or oats.
Avoid Sugar and Processed Foods – Get Rid of the Junk! Eat Real Food	Sugar spikes insulin levels, leading to fat storage, especially around the abdomen. Processed foods are often packed with hidden sugars, additives and preservatives that can disrupt hormones and even trigger menopause symptoms like fatigue, bloating, hot flashes and mood swings. If you can't make it in your kitchen or if the ingredients list includes things you don't recognise or can't pronounce, you probably shouldn't be eating it. Stick to real, whole foods that nourish your body.	Action Step: Limit sugary snacks, fizzy drinks and all processed foods. When craving something sweet, opt for low-sugar fruits like berries, kiwi, grapefruit and green apples, or use natural sweeteners like cinnamon or vanilla to enhance flavour without the sugar spike.

Use Smaller Plates	Portion sizes have grown over the years and so have our plates! I still have my granny's dinner plates and they are much smaller than the ones we use today.	Action Step: Swap your regular dinner plate for a smaller one to naturally and effortlessly reduce portion sizes.
Drink water	It helps control hunger and supports metabolism.	Action Step: Aim for around 8 glasses of water daily and drink a glass before meals to prevent overeating.
Plan Balanced Meals for Sustainable Weight Loss	A balanced plate with protein, healthy fats, fibre and complex carbs keeps hunger in check and energy steady. For weight loss, focus on non-starchy vegetables as the foundation of your meal. Think leafy greens, peppers, broccoli, cauliflower, courgette, asparagus and mushrooms. Then, add protein such as	Action Step: Fill half your plate with non-starchy vegetables, a quarter with protein, and a small portion of starchy vegetables like sweet potato, squash, or quinoa if needed. If weight loss is your goal, keep starchy vegetables and whole grains to a minimum, prioritising protein, fats, and fibre-rich vegetables for sustainable results.

	chicken, fish, tofu, eggs, or lentils, along with healthy fats like olive oil, avocado, nuts, or seeds.	
Limit Alcohol	Alcohol is high in empty calories and can disrupt sleep and hormone balance. If you choose to drink, opt for options with the least sugar to minimise the impact, e.g. dry white wines, or dry sparkling wines. Looking at the labels and choosing the ones with the least sugar and alcohol is a good start.	Action Step: Reduce alcohol intake or save it for special occasions. Opt for dry white wine or clear spirits and limit to one serving to support your health goals.
Increase Omega-3s	Omega-3s reduce inflammation and help maintain muscle mass. For those following a vegan lifestyle, there are excellent plant-based sources of omega-3s, such as flaxseeds, chia	Action Step: Eat fatty fish like salmon, or for a plant-based option, include foods like flaxseeds or take an algal oil supplement.

	seeds, hemp seeds and walnuts. Algal oil, derived from marine algae, is also a highly effective vegan alternative to fish oil.	
Eat Mindfully	Eating slowly, paying attention to hunger cues can help prevent overeating.	Action Step: Sit down for meals, chew thoroughly and avoid distractions like TV or phones.
Shorten your Eating Window	Reducing the hours you eat each day can give your body more time to rest and digest, improving metabolism.	Action Step: Try intermittent fasting by closing your eating window to 10-12 hours during the day, such as from 8 AM to 6 PM (see more information on this in chapter 3).

"You don't need to count calories or starve yourself to maintain a healthy weight during menopause. By nourishing your body with real, nutritious foods and focusing on getting enough sleep and exercise, you can avoid unwanted weight gain and feel good about yourself again"

Tea

I am a lover of tea. It must be my Britishness, one tea that I discovered a few years ago called Pu-erh (yes I know it's a funny one to pronounce!) is not only delicious but has potential weight loss benefits. It is a fermented tea from China's Yunnan province. A study published in the Journal of Food Measurement and Characterization found that citrus Pu-erh tea extract intake may stimulate digestion and reduce the release of free fatty acids, suggesting a potential role in managing fat digestion and absorption. A study in the European Journal of Nutrition reported that theabrownin, a component of Pu-erh tea, may influence lipid metabolism, suppress body weight gain and improve insulin sensitivity in obese mice. And if that is not enough it has been shown to suppress appetite, helping to reduce overall calorie intake. It's not a miracle cure but another thing we can add to our daily routine and have in your toolkit. Incorporating Pu-erh tea into your daily routine may offer additional support in your weight loss journey alongside balanced nutrition and a healthy lifestyle.

Testosterone and Weight Management in Women

Testosterone isn't just a male hormone; women also produce small amounts, and it plays a vital role in regulating muscle mass, fat distribution and energy levels. As we age, testosterone levels decline. This decrease can lead to a reduction in muscle mass, making it harder to maintain a healthy weight. Building muscle through strength training and maintaining balanced hormone levels can help support your metabolism and prevent weight gain.

Research suggests that keeping testosterone levels balanced through lifestyle adjustments like exercise, good sleep and stress management can aid in healthier weight maintenance.

Beyond Food: Uncovering the Hidden Factors Affecting Weight in Menopause

When it comes to weight management, it's not just about food. There are other important factors that are often overlooked. First, let's talk about stress. Yes, good old stress that so many of us seem to be battling these days. I'll look deeper into this in chapter 8, but for now, let's focus on how stress affects your weight.

I've seen how stress management is key to successful weight loss. "Why?", you may ask. The reason lies with the stress hormone cortisol. Chronic stress elevates cortisol levels and this promotes fat storage, especially around the tummy. High cortisol also increases cravings for sugary and processed foods, which makes weight loss even harder. Finding realistic ways to manage stress is essential if you want to lose weight and keep it off.

Poor sleep, another common issue, can also wreak havoc on your hormones and your weight. When you don't get good quality sleep, your levels of leptin (the hormone that signals fullness) drop, while ghrelin (the hormone that triggers hunger) rises. This imbalance can lead to overeating and cravings, making it much harder to maintain your weight. Research shows that women in menopause who experience sleep disruptions are more likely to gain weight. For practical tips on how to improve your sleep, head to chapter 6.

We also tend to lose muscle mass as we age. While this is a natural part of getting older, it's important to remember that muscle is highly metabolically active. In other words, it burns calories, even when you're sitting on the sofa watching your favourite TV program. Muscles are often referred to as the organs of longevity and the longer we keep them, the better it is for every aspect of our health, including weight management. Think of muscle as your body's furnace. The more muscle you have, the more calories you burn. To learn more about maintaining muscle mass, check out chapter 9. Eating enough protein and doing weight-bearing exercises you enjoy are some of the best ways to keep your muscles happy and healthy.

Menopause can also make you more prone to insulin resistance as your oestrogen levels decline. This means your body struggles to process glucose efficiently, which can lead to more fat being stored, especially around the tummy. You might have heard it called the 'meno belly' or muffin top! Balancing your meals and managing your blood sugar levels, as we talked about in chapter 3, are crucial steps in maintaining or losing weight if that's your goal.

Impact of Environmental Toxins (Endocrine Disruptors)

Another factor that often flies under the radar is the role of environmental toxins. Certain chemicals found in plastics, cleaning products and cosmetics (like BPA and phthalates) can mimic hormones and disrupt your endocrine system, making it harder to maintain a healthy weight. These endocrine disruptors can interfere with hormone balance, promoting fat storage and contributing to other health issues.

Lastly, let's not forget the emotional side of things. How you feel emotionally can have a big impact on your weight and eating habits. If you're feeling down or depressed, it's easy to turn to food for comfort, which can make weight loss more challenging. Acknowledging this emotional connection and finding ways to support your mental well-being is a key part of the bigger picture for managing your weight.

The Buzz Around Weight Loss Injections: What You Need to Know

It can be incredibly frustrating to manage weight during menopause, especially with all the hormonal shifts that make it feel like an uphill battle. This chapter wouldn't be complete without acknowledging the growing interest in GLP-1 agonist medications, which have received a lot of attention over the past year as tools for weight management. These injectable medications are often viewed as a possible solution for women in menopause, but it's important to take a closer look at what they actually offer and to consider the full picture before deciding if they're right for you.

How They Work

These medications, known as Glucagon-Like Peptide-1 (GLP-1) receptor agonists, were originally developed to help manage type 2 diabetes but have gained attention for their role in weight loss. GLP-1 is a natural hormone released in the gut that helps regulate appetite, digestion and blood sugar levels. These medications mimic the effects of GLP-1, leading to several key benefits for weight management:

Appetite Regulation – They signal to the brain that you're full, helping to reduce food intake and prevent overeating.

Slower Digestion – They delay the emptying of food from the stomach, keeping you fuller for longer and helping to stabilise blood sugar levels.

Craving Control – By interacting with hunger-related hormones, they can help reduce cravings for sugary or processed foods.

Improved Blood Sugar Management – By enhancing insulin release and reducing glucose spikes after meals, they can help prevent the blood sugar crashes that often lead to energy dips and cravings.

The upside

For women in perimenopause and menopause, when hormonal shifts make weight management more challenging, these injections can be a helpful tool. Research shows they can support meaningful weight loss, improve metabolic health, and reduce the risk of conditions like heart disease and type 2 diabetes.

The downsides to consider

However, these medications are not without drawbacks. More research is needed, and common side effects include nausea, digestive discomfort and fatigue. There's also been growing conversation around what's been coined "Ozempic face," a term used by plastic surgeons to describe the sagging or hollowed appearance that can occur with rapid weight loss. While this isn't directly caused by the medication itself, it highlights the importance of gradual and sustainable weight loss, especially for women already dealing with changes in skin elasticity during menopause.

Another significant consideration is that these injections often need to be taken long-term to maintain results. Some studies have shown that once the medication is stopped, weight lost is often regained. Additionally, these drugs are still relatively new and we really don't know their long-term effects yet. More research is needed to fully understand their safety and effectiveness over time, making it important to approach them with caution.

Natural Ways to Boost GLP-1

- Eat protein at every meal.

- Add fibre from veggies, seeds, and wholegrains.

- Move daily – even just a walk after meals.

- Prioritise sleep to balance hunger hormones.

- Stay hydrated, especially before meals.

Looking at the Bigger Picture

While weight loss injections may offer a useful tool for women struggling with stubborn weight gain during menopause, they are not a replacement for the foundational habits of good health. Sustainable weight management is deeply tied to balanced eating, regular movement, stress management and overall lifestyle. These injections, if used, should complement, not replace, those essential elements.

Is it Right for You?

If you're considering weight loss injections, it's crucial to consult with a trusted healthcare professional to assess whether they're appropriate for your needs. These medications were not designed as a quick fix for losing a few kilograms but as part of a comprehensive approach to health. They should not replace sustainable lifestyle habits.

Supportive Treatments for Weight Management and Body Confidence

Unfortunately, as we have discussed there is no quick fix for weight loss. There isn't just one thing we can do that will solve everything. Looking at what you eat, managing your stress, and focusing on your lifestyle habits like exercise and sleep are the foundations for long-term weight management. However, I have seen in my many years of working with clients as a beauty therapist that professional salon treatments can play a part in your weight loss journey. Aesthetic treatments can complement a holistic approach to feeling better and more confident during your weight loss journey, particularly in areas like skin appearance, skin tightening, reducing cellulite, enhancing lymphatic drainage and promoting better body contouring and body image. This can motivate you and make you feel more confident as you work towards your weight loss goals.

Here are some treatments that are backed by research. I have worked with many of these treatments and seen good results over time. Always go to a registered aesthetician (posh word for beauty therapist) that is trained in these treatments. Do your homework first and find a good reputable clinic.

Treatments		
Name	How it works	Effectiveness
Cryolipolysis	Cryolipolysis is a non-invasive fat-freezing (I love that expression fat freezing it sounds too good to be true doesn't it!) technique that targets and can help to eliminate stubborn fat cells without surgery. It is most effective on localised fat areas such as the abdomen, thighs and those love handles. You would normally need a course of several treatments.	Studies have shown that CoolSculpting can reduce fat by up to 25% in treated areas after a single session, though it requires a few weeks to see full results. It's particularly effective for body contouring rather than overall weight loss.

You may have heard of cryotherapy which is not the same as Cryolipolysis. Both treatments use cold but serve very different purposes. Cryotherapy typically takes place in a chamber where your body is briefly exposed to extremely cold temperatures to reduce inflammation, improve circulation and boost overall wellness. It's often used by athletes for |

		recovery or for general health, not specifically for fat loss.
		Cryolipolysis, like 'CoolSculpting', is a targeted fat reduction treatment that uses a machine to freeze fat cells in specific areas (like the belly or thighs). Your body naturally eliminates these fat cells over time, making Cryolipolysis a cosmetic procedure focused on body contouring.
Radiofrequency Skin Tightening	Radiofrequency (RF) skin tightening uses heat energy to penetrate the skin's deeper layers, stimulating collagen production. This process helps tighten and firm the skin, especially in areas where sagging may	While RF treatments don't directly target fat loss, they are effective for improving skin elasticity and appearance, making them ideal for body contouring after weight loss.

	occur after weight loss.	
Ultrasound Cavitation Treatments	Ultrasound treatments use low-frequency sound waves to break down fat cells. These fat cells are then naturally processed and eliminated by the body through the lymphatic system.	While not designed for significant weight loss, ultrasound treatments can reduce fat deposits in targeted areas like the abdomen or thighs, helping with body contouring. Multiple sessions may be required for noticeable results.

Gentle Therapies That Support Weight Loss

When it comes to weight loss, it's not just about diet and exercise. When combined with a healthy lifestyle, there are also some incredible natural treatments that can work alongside these efforts to support your body and help you achieve your goals in a more holistic and balanced way.

Lymphatic Drainage Massage

This manual massage technique is a great way to stimulate the lymphatic system. It helps reduce water retention and can help beat that bloating feeling, which can make you feel lighter and look and feel slimmer. Not only that, but it also supports your body's detoxification process, giving you an extra boost.

Body Wraps

If you're looking for a quick way to tighten and tone your skin, body wraps are a good option. Using herbal, mineral, or clay-based wraps, these treatments temporarily reduce water retention and firm the skin. It's a great confidence boost when you're feeling puffy or bloated.

Acupuncture

Acupuncture works by balancing your energy flow and can be a helpful tool in regulating your metabolism. It's also known to reduce cravings and improve digestion which can be helpful when trying to manage your weight naturally.

Dry Brushing

All you need is a brush! This simple yet effective exfoliating technique can do wonders for your circulation. I absolutely love dry brushing and make it part of my morning routine before I shower. It's so easy, takes just a few minutes and delivers amazing benefits.

Dry brushing stimulates blood flow, encourages lymphatic drainage and supports your body's natural detoxification process, which can enhance your weight loss efforts over time. It's also fantastic for improving the appearance of cellulite, a concern many of us notice more as we transition into menopause. Give it a try and see how this small habit can make a big difference.

Infrared Sauna

Using an infrared sauna regularly (3-4 times per week) can help with weight loss by promoting deep detoxification and burning calories.

Studies show that infrared saunas can aid in reducing body fat by increasing heart rate and metabolism, similar to the effects of moderate exercise. They're also fantastic for stress reduction, which we know is crucial for managing weight. Infrared saunas penetrate deeper into the skin compared to traditional saunas, improving circulation and giving your metabolism a gentle boost.

Stress Reduction Techniques

Finally, let's not forget the importance of managing stress during menopause. High stress leads to increased cortisol levels, which can make weight loss more difficult. Incorporating stress-reducing practices like massage, meditation, or yoga helps lower cortisol, reduce cravings and balance your metabolism.

Each of these treatments can be powerful on their own, but when combined with a healthy lifestyle, they can amplify your weight loss efforts. The key is consistency and finding what works best for you.

Actionable Weight Management Wellness Tips

Drink a Glass of Water Before Every Meal: This can help control your appetite and support digestion, making it easier to manage portion size.

Move for 10 Minutes After Each Meal: A short walk or gentle movement after eating helps boost digestion and blood sugar balance helping to support your weight loss goals.

Common Mistakes with Weight Loss

In my clinic, I often see women doing their very best but still feeling stuck — not because they're not trying hard enough, but because certain habits or assumptions are unknowingly working against them. Here are some of the most common weight loss mistakes I see time and time again during perimenopause and menopause. Awareness is the first step to change!

- Relying on crash diets
- Underestimating the impact of stress
- Not getting enough protein
- Ignoring sleep
- Expecting quick results
- Eating for emotional comfort
- Not being honest with yourself about what you're eating
- Portion control
- Drinking alcohol regularly
- Not moving enough
- Thinking you can eat more after exercising
- Eating sugary foods at breakfast
- Lack of consistency
- Falling for food saboteurs
- Eating while distracted by your electronic devices
- Snacking too much like a grazer
- Eating low-fat foods

- Over-reliance on processed 'health' foods
- Skipping meals and then overeating later
- Not drinking enough water
- Ignoring fibre intake
- Focusing only on the scales
- Underestimating hidden sugars
- Not planning meals in advance
- Not Strength Training
- Using artificial sweeteners thinking they're better
- Drinking your calories
- Not managing blood sugar levels

Supplements to Consider for Supporting Menopausal Weight Loss

- **Berberine** – Supports blood sugar balance, insulin sensitivity, and metabolism. Use with professional guidance.

- **Ashwagandha** (KSM-66) – Helps manage cortisol and stress-related weight gain; supports thyroid health.

- **Magnesium** (Glycinate or Citrate) – Aids energy, blood sugar balance, and reduces stress-related cravings.

- **Alpha Lipoic Acid** (ALA) – Promotes blood sugar control, liver detox support, and metabolic health.

- **Inositol** (myo- and d-chiro blend) – Balances insulin, supports weight management, and hormonal regulation.

- **Protein powder** if you find it hard to get enough protein in your diet.

Three Quick Wins

1. Use Smaller Plates - Shrink your portion sizes without even noticing. Smaller plates can help you eat less while still feeling satisfied.

2. Add Protein to Every Meal - Protein helps curb cravings, supports lean muscle and keeps you feeling fuller for longer all essential for steady weight loss.

3. Cut Out Alcohol for 2 Weeks - Alcohol slows fat burning, affects sleep and adds empty calories. Take a break for two weeks and see how it impacts your waistline and energy.

5 HOW TO BOOST YOUR ENERGY AND STOP FEELING EXHAUSTED!

"Almost everything will work again if you unplug it for a few minutes... including you."

Anne Lamott

Five Things You'll Learn in this Chapter:

- **Why your energy dips** during perimenopause
- How hormonal changes affect your **energy, sleep and mood**
- **Practical nutrition strategies** to help you feel more energised
- **Lifestyle tweaks** that support better sleep, focus and stamina
- **Simple at-home and salon rituals** that can help you recharge

Are you the "constantly-on-the-go woman," charging around juggling a busy home life, a career and trying to push through your never-ending to-do list? As women, we tend to be the carers, always looking after everyone else and putting ourselves last. Let's be honest we often come at the very bottom of that list. And here's the truth: your to-do list will never be done because you are always adding to it. If you're waiting to finish that list before you start looking after yourself, you'll be waiting forever. The to-do list can wait, you, however, cannot. You should be at the very top of that list.

In your 20s and 30s, this constant rush of daily life seemed manageable. Sure, there were moments of tiredness, like when you'd had a late night or one too many glasses of wine, but somehow you'd bounce back. Fast forward to your 40s and things feel different. Perimenopause starts creeping in and suddenly your energy levels don't seem to stretch as far. The word exhaustion, once just something you heard other women talk about, suddenly becomes an all-too-familiar reality.

In this chapter, we're going to talk about why you feel so much more tired now and more importantly, what you can do about it. I'll dig into the hormonal changes that are happening in your body and uncover what's contributing to that "always tired" feeling.

"Exhaustion isn't a badge of honour, it's your body waving a red flag, begging you to slow down and recharge."

Alison Bladh

But don't worry, I promise the strategies I'm about to share won't take up much brain power or add stress to your life and make you feel even more tired. I can imagine you've got enough on your plate as it is. This is about helping you reclaim your energy in a way that feels simple, practical and most importantly doable. You deserve to feel like yourself again and this chapter will show you how.

> As women, we're always taking care of everyone else, but when was the last time you cared for yourself? The to-do list will never end, but your energy will unless you start making yourself a priority.

The Energy Dips – Why Does This Happen?

Does everything suddenly feel like an uphill battle? You're not alone. Fatigue during perimenopause and menopause can manifest in many ways, and it's not just about feeling tired, it's a whole-body experience that can make even the simplest tasks feel overwhelming.

Here are some common signs of fatigue that might be showing up for you:

Physical Fatigue: Feeling drained, like your body just doesn't have the energy to keep up with your daily routine.

Mental Fog: Trouble concentrating, forgetfulness, or difficulty processing information often called "brain fog."

Irritability: Feeling more easily frustrated or annoyed, even by small things (I can certainly relate to this one!).

Sleep Disruptions: Struggling to fall asleep, stay asleep, or waking up still feeling tired.

Muscle Weakness: Heaviness or a lack of strength in your limbs, making movement feel like a chore.

Headaches: Persistent fatigue can sometimes trigger headaches or migraines.

Emotional Distress: Anxiety, mood swings, or feeling overwhelmed often accompany exhaustion.

Decreased Motivation: A lack of drive or interest in tasks, even ones you used to enjoy.

Low Immunity: Feeling run down or more prone to catching colds or infections.

Digestive Issues: Bloating, upset stomach, or irregular digestion that leaves you feeling uncomfortable and sluggish.

Sound familiar? So why does this happen? The hormonal shifts during menopause are at the root of this energy dip, disrupting the delicate balance in your body and making even simple tasks feel harder.

The Reasons Behind the Energy Dips

Fluctuating Oestrogen Levels

Oestrogen helps regulate serotonin, the "feel-good" hormone that influences mood and energy. When oestrogen levels drop, serotonin dips too, leading to low energy, fatigue and even feelings of sadness.

Heavy Periods

During perimenopause, periods can become heavier and more unpredictable. Sometimes you might even have two in one month. This can result in significant iron loss, potentially causing anaemia. If your iron levels drop, you might feel completely drained and experience symptoms like palpitations, headaches, or a sore tongue.

Declining Progesterone

Progesterone is known for promoting relaxation and restful sleep. As levels decline, sleep can become more fragmented, leaving you tired no matter how long you spend in bed.

Lower Testosterone

Testosterone isn't just a male hormone; it plays a key role in maintaining muscle strength and energy in women too. When testosterone levels drop, physical tiredness and weakness can set in, making even simple tasks feel more exhausting.

Sleep Disruptions

Hot flushes, night sweats and insomnia are common during menopause. Poor sleep quality not only leaves you tired but also affects your ability to concentrate, creating a vicious cycle of exhaustion.

Blood Sugar Fluctuations

Hormonal changes can impact how your body regulates blood sugar levels. This can lead to energy crashes, particularly after eating, making it difficult to stay alert and focused throughout the day.

Nutritional Deficiencies

Nutritional deficiencies are a common but overlooked cause of fatigue during menopause. Key nutrients needed for energy production include B vitamins (especially B12 and B6), magnesium, vitamin D, zinc and coenzyme Q10. These nutrients play vital roles in supporting your metabolism, reducing tiredness, and helping your cells produce energy efficiently.

If you're feeling constantly fatigued, consider testing for deficiencies with your healthcare provider. Replenishing these nutrients through diet or supplements can make a big difference to how energised you feel day to day.

The Stress of Life

Let's face it this stage of life often comes with additional responsibilities, from work and family to caregiving. Combined with hormonal changes, these pressures can leave you feeling more fatigued and less resilient.

Thyroid Issues

Perimenopause can increase the risk of developing thyroid problems, which can slow metabolism and cause sluggishness. If you're feeling persistently tired, it might be worth checking your thyroid function.

Cognitive Fatigue (" Brain Fog")

Alongside physical fatigue, many women experience cognitive issues like forgetfulness and difficulty focusing. Declining oestrogen levels disrupt neurotransmitters like serotonin and dopamine, which influence both mood and energy. (We'll dive deeper into this in chapter 7 when we explore brain health and mental clarity.)

> *"Women need solitude in order to find again the true essence of themselves."*
>
> **Anne Morrow Lindbergh**

A Path to More Energy

By understanding the reasons behind this energy dip, you're already on the first step to addressing it. The good news? You don't have to accept this as your new normal. In the rest of this chapter, we'll explore practical ways to boost your energy and help you feel more like yourself again.

What Can We Do?

Now that you understand why your energy levels might be dipping, let's talk about what you can do to start feeling better. These are simple, practical steps that can really make a difference. Think of this as a toolkit of simple things you can do to support your energy.

Nutrition-Based Ways to Boost Energy

- Drink at least 2 litres of water daily to stay hydrated and support cellular energy production

- Eat a protein-rich breakfast to stabilise blood sugar and support alertness throughout the day

- Include healthy fats like avocado, nuts, seeds and olive oil to fuel your brain and hormones

- Avoid sugary snacks that cause energy crashes — choose slow-release carbs instead

- Balance every meal with protein, healthy fats and fibre to avoid blood sugar dips

- Consider closing your eating window to support digestion and mitochondrial function

- Limit alcohol and caffeine, especially in the afternoon, to avoid disrupted sleep and fatigue

- Support your gut health with fermented foods and prebiotic fibre, energy starts in the gut

- Eat magnesium-rich foods (like leafy greens and pumpkin seeds) to reduce tiredness

- Check for nutrient deficiencies (especially B12, iron, vitamin D and magnesium) even mild deficiencies can leave you feeling drained

- Add adaptogens like ashwagandha or rhodiola (with guidance) to support energy and stress resilience

- Don't skip meals — regular eating supports stable energy and hormone balance

Lifestyle-Based Ways to Boost Energy

- Moving your body daily, even a 10-minute walk boosts circulation and lifts your mood

- Using a stand-up desk or take regular stretch breaks if you sit for long periods

- Getting outside in natural daylight every morning to reset your body clock and lift your energy naturally

- Taking short breaks throughout the day to avoid burnout — even a few deep breaths can help

- Managing stress with calming practices like yoga, meditation, or simple breathing exercises

- Prioritising quality sleep, aim for 7–9 hours and keep a consistent bedtime

- Laughing often. It's a natural stress reliever and boosts your energy instantly

- Meeting friends regularly. Social connection is vital for emotional and physical energy

- Doing things that bring you joy, pleasure and purpose are powerful energisers

- Limiting screen time before bed to support melatonin production and restful sleep

- Trying contrast showers (alternating hot and cold) in the morning to invigorate your nervous system

- Practicing gratitude or journaling in the evening to calm your mind and promote restorative sleep

---

Have You Heard of Laughter Yoga?

Laughter Yoga combines deep breathing with intentional laughter to boost energy and mood. It might feel odd at first. I've tried it and it definitely felt a bit strange! But once you get going, it's brilliant. Even fake laughter boosts endorphins, lowers stress hormones and lifts your energy. Give it a go, it really works!

What Your Day Could Look Like to Boost Energy

Here is a simple, structured guide to fuel your body, stay active and maintain steady energy levels throughout the day.

Time	Action
7:00 AM	Drink a big glass of water to rehydrate after sleep.
7:30 AM	Eat a protein-rich breakfast to stabilise blood sugar.
9:00 AM	Get outside for natural daylight and take a 5-minute walk.
10:30 AM	Stand up and stretch to reduce stiffness and improve circulation.
12:00 PM	Take short breaks to move, refresh, drink a glass of water.
12:30 PM	Eat a balanced lunch with protein, healthy fats and veggies.
3:00 PM	Have a healthy snack (avoid sugary foods to prevent energy crashes).
4:00 PM	Do light movement or exercise for 10 minutes to recharge.
6:00 PM	Manage stress with mindfulness, deep breathing, or journaling.
6:30 PM	Enjoy a nourishing dinner with protein, healthy fats and veggies.
8:00 PM	Close your eating window after dinner to support digestion and metabolic balance.
9:30 PM	Create a relaxing bedtime routine to promote restful sleep.

Creatine: Your secret weapon for energy

Creatine isn't just for bodybuilders, it's a supplement for women looking to boost energy and support their overall health. Found naturally in the body, creatine plays a key role in producing adenosine triphosphate (ATP), the energy your cells rely on to keep you going. As we age, our muscle mass and energy levels naturally decline, and creatine can help bridge that gap. It's especially useful if you're feeling fatigued or struggling to maintain strength during exercise. Studies even suggest it may support brain health, making it a great all-rounder for boosting both physical and mental energy.

I would recommend when buying creatine, look for creatine monohydrate, the most researched and effective form. Choose a high-quality, pure product without unnecessary additives and as always, check with your healthcare provider to ensure it's right for you.

"Exhaustion isn't just tiredness, it's your body pleading for rest and the chance to recharge"

Reclaim Your Energy:
At-Home Rituals and Salon Treatments

I know we all hear so much about self-care these days which, don't get me wrong, is great and it certainly can help you regain some energy when you are feeling exhausted, but the thing is it's not enough just to grab a few minutes on a Saturday while shopping, cleaning the house and feeding your family members. During menopause you really need to ramp up your 'me' time. Putting yourself first means you will have more energy and feel happier in yourself. I am realistic and understand you are constantly on the go! Most women do not have time for long fancy selfcare rituals that are wonderful but are not accessible or sustainable for everyone.

Spending a weekend at a spa with your girlfriend is such a wonderful way to help reclaim your energy levels. Spending an evening talking with your friends laughing and joking is so rejuvenating. I find laughter is powerful. It revives you and there is plenty of research to back this up. Not only does it boost your energy levels, but it helps reduce stress and it also feels great to laugh. I don't know what you think, but I feel we don't laugh as much as we used to. So, let's talk about what at home rituals or treatments you can use to boost your energy and stop feeling exhausted all the time.

My beauty therapy side always wants to jump in here, so I can't resist sharing some professional treatments that can really help with boosting energy and tackling that tired, run-down feeling. There's something so uplifting about taking a little time to focus on yourself and feel truly rejuvenated, I just love that word! These treatments aren't just about looking good, they're about giving you that much-needed boost to feel better inside and out. Let's explore some options that can work wonders.

Putting yourself first isn't selfish, it's necessary. During menopause, your energy is precious and you deserve to recharge in ways that work for you. Whether it's a simple stretch, a refreshing facial mist, or a much-needed massage, every little bit counts. You're constantly caring for others now it's time to care for yourself.

Massage: Your Menopause Best Friend

Massage is one of the simplest yet most powerful ways to relax, recharge and support your body through perimenopause and menopause. Think of it as a reset button helping to ease tension, boost circulation and calm the nervous system when everything feels overwhelming.

If you've never had a massage before, a classic Swedish massage is a great place to start. It's deeply relaxing, helps with muscle aches, and encourages better sleep. Or, if you're looking for a quick pick-me-up, a facial massage can work wonders reducing muscle tension, giving your skin a natural energy lift, and helping you feel refreshed.

Whatever type you choose, regular massage can be a game-changer in helping you feel balanced, calm, and more in tune with your body during this transition.

Then we have aromatherapy massage which is known for its stress-relieving and energy-boosting effects. Essential oils like lavender, lemon, eucalyptus, rosemary and peppermint are commonly used to reduce fatigue and improve mood. Research suggests that aromatherapy can help regulate cortisol levels, improve sleep and reduce stress, all of which contribute to higher energy levels.

Reiki is an energy healing practice that has been found to reduce stress and boost feelings of vitality. While the research is more limited, some studies suggest that Reiki can help menopausal women feel more balanced and energised by reducing stress and promoting relaxation.

If you like saunas, infrared saunas are a great thing to do. infrared saunas provide heat that penetrates deep into the body, helping to detoxify, improve circulation and reduce stress. Research has shown that regular use can improve energy levels, reduce fatigue and enhance overall well-being, especially for women experiencing menopause-related exhaustion.

Reflexology has been around for many years and has been shown to help promote energy levels and balance in the body. It is performed on the feet where different pressure points that correspond to different areas on your body, are stimulated.

Gua Sha massage is another option worth considering. This ancient technique uses smooth tools to gently scrape the skin, improving circulation, releasing tension, and promoting lymphatic drainage. It's deeply relaxing and rejuvenating, a menopausal woman's best-kept secret for feeling recharged. You can buy these tools and use them at home on yourself.

"You've spent years taking care of everyone else. Now it's your turn. Reclaim your energy, not by waiting for a weekend spa trip, but in the little moments, right at home. Small steps can make a big difference."

Salon treatments aren't everyone's cup of tea. Maybe you're thinking, I'd love to, but I just don't have the time, or perhaps it feels a bit too indulgent for you right now. The good news is, there are plenty of things you can do at home to help with exhaustion and boost your energy levels. Here are a few of my favourite recharge rituals to get you started.

Recharge Rituals	
What	**Action**
Cold Face Splash. Cryotherapy-Inspired. Splashing cold water on your face is a quick and easy way to perk up. It stimulates circulation, boosts your mood and helps reset your nervous system.	Splash your face with cold water in the morning, or use a cool cloth from the fridge whenever you need a boost.
DIY Aromatherapy Shower. Add a few drops of citrus or peppermint essential oil to a flannel or use a pre-made shower	Avoid putting oils directly on the shower floor to prevent slipping. Instead, drop them onto a flannel or use a safe steamer

steamer. The steam helps lift your mood and boost your energy.	product.
Facial Mist. Using a refreshing mist with peppermint or citrus essential oils can invigorate the senses and energise your mood.	Keep a small spray in your handbag or on your desk and use it anytime you need a little lift.
10-Minute Stretching Routine. Stretching boosts circulation and releases muscle tension.	Schedule mini stretch breaks into your day, neck rolls, shoulder shrugs and gentle twists do wonders.
Sheet Mask Cool Down. A cooling face mask from the fridge not only revives tired skin but also gives you a midday mood lift.	Keep one in the fridge and use it when you can for a relaxing reset.
Body Brushing. Dry brushing before your morning shower wakes up your skin and your senses. I do this every day, it's one of my favourite ways to start the day.	Use a soft natural bristle brush, working in upward strokes towards your heart.
Cold Showers. A quick cold blast at the end of your shower can boost circulation and alertness.	Finish with 30–60 seconds of cold water. Start small and build up.
Gua Sha or Jade Roller Facial.	Apply facial oil and gently roll

These tools stimulate the lymphatic system, reduce puffiness and help you feel fresher.	upward across your cheeks, jawline and forehead for five minutes.
Grounding (Earthing). Walking barefoot on natural surfaces like grass, soil or sand can help reset your nervous system, reduce inflammation and support deeper sleep, all crucial for energy.	Spend 10–15 minutes barefoot outdoors each day, ideally in the morning for an added dose of daylight.
Evening Magnesium Bath. Magnesium is essential for energy metabolism, stress relief and muscle relaxation and many women are low in it. A warm bath with Epsom salts is soothing and replenishing.	Add 1–2 cups of magnesium flakes to your bath and soak for 20 minutes a few evenings a week.
Binaural Beats or Sound Therapy. Listening to low-frequency binaural beats has been shown to reduce fatigue and stress while enhancing focus and calm.	Put on your headphones and listen to a 10–15 minute binaural beat session when you feel tired, particularly in the afternoon.
Alternate Nostril Breathing (Nadi Shodhana). This yogic breathwork technique balances	Try 3 minutes of alternate nostril breathing in the morning or mid-afternoon slump.

both hemispheres of the brain and improves oxygenation. It's energising but calming too perfect for fatigue that feels mental and physical.	
Protein + Adaptogen Latte. Combine a scoop of good quality protein powder with adaptogens like maca, ashwagandha or reishi into a warm drink. Adaptogens help regulate stress hormones, while the protein supports blood sugar balance.	Replace your second coffee with a protein adaptogen latte and note the difference in energy and calmness.

If you love a bit of pampering (and who doesn't?), salon treatments can play a surprisingly effective role in helping you feel energised. These aren't just about looking good, they're about helping you feel good, too.

As a beauty therapist, I've worked with many clients who come in feeling run-down and leave with renewed energy and confidence. Whether it's through touch, scent, heat or healing techniques, the power of professional treatments to help you reset shouldn't be underestimated.

Supplements to Consider for Energy Support

- **Magnesium (Glycinate or Malate)** – Supports energy production, muscle function, and nervous system regulation. Malate is especially helpful for fatigue.

- **Vitamin B Complex (Activated)** – Essential for energy metabolism, stress response and red blood cell production. Look for B6 (P-5-P), B12 (methylcobalamin), and folate (5-MTHF).

- **Iron (Bisglycinate)** – If you're low in iron, it can severely impact energy levels. Choose a gentle, absorbable form and only supplement if deficiency is confirmed.

- **CoQ10 (Ubiquinol)** – Supports mitochondrial function and cellular energy production. Especially useful for women over 40, as levels naturally decline with age.

- **Vitamin D3** – Low vitamin D is associated with fatigue, low mood and poor immune resilience. Best taken with K2 for absorption and bone support.

- **Adaptogens (e.g. Rhodiola, Eleuthero, Ashwagandha)** – Help balance cortisol, reduce fatigue and support resilience to stress-related energy crashes.

- **Alpha Lipoic Acid (ALA)** – Supports energy, blood sugar balance and antioxidant protection.

Three Quick Wins

1. Stand up and do 10 heel raises - Lifting your heels off the ground and lowering them slowly gets your circulation moving. Great if you've been sitting too long and need a quick pick-me-up.

2. Rub peppermint oil on your wrists - The scent can refresh your senses, clear your head and make you feel more awake perfect for that mid-afternoon slump. (Just make sure it's diluted in a carrier oil!).

3. Look out of a window and blink slowly 10 times - It calms your nervous system, gives your eyes a break from screens and helps reset mental fatigue.

6 SLEEP LIKE A QUEEN

"Sleep isn't a luxury, it's the foundation of how you think, feel and function. Prioritising it is one of the most powerful things you can do for your hormones, your skin and your sanity."

Alison Bladh

Five Things You'll Learn in this Chapter:

- **Why sleep becomes more challenging** during perimenopause and menopause and what your hormones have to do with it.

- **The link between poor sleep and skin health** and how beauty really does start with a good night's rest.

- **The surprising truth about "chasing sleep"** and why letting go might actually help you sleep better.

- **How your nutrition, stress, and evening habits** could be secretly sabotaging your rest.

- **Simple, effective rituals and tools** to help you fall asleep, stay asleep and wake up feeling like yourself again.

Imagine waking up refreshed, with glowing skin and a sense of calm that carries you through the day. Quality sleep isn't just a dream. It's a powerful tool for navigating menopause with energy, calm and a sense of control. That said, I'm certainly not claiming it's easy. Sleep often becomes a struggle as we hit our mid-40s and perimenopause sneaks in.

I know this struggle first-hand. I call it the '3 o'clock club.'

How many women around the world lie awake in the early hours of the morning, wide-eyed and restless, thanks to the hormonal changes of menopause? A friend of mine even started a Facebook group called the '3am club', which quickly grew in popularity. Not that I'm saying scrolling on your phone in the middle of the night will help you drift back to sleep. It definitely won't!

I've become super protective of my sleep, especially as it's become worse with age. I just don't function well without a solid seven to eight hours of rest. I stick to a routine, going to bed at the same time every evening, around 9.30pm and waking up at 6.30am. One thing that's really helped me is avoiding devices at least an hour before bed. Turn off anything that over-stimulates your brain and give yourself the chance to wind down properly, it makes all the difference and yes, your phone does have an off button!

Even the soundest sleepers can find themselves battling restless nights during this time, waking up drained and defeated. It's a frustrating cycle that affects every aspect of life, but understanding why it happens is the first step to reclaiming those precious hours of rest.

I really value the insights of Dr. Sara Gottfried, a leading women's health expert, who emphasises, "Sleep is the foundation of hormonal balance and without it, everything from your mood to your metabolism suffers." This is especially true during menopause, when quality sleep is vital for stabilising hormones, boosting energy, improving mood and even supporting skin health.

In this chapter, we'll uncover practical ways to harness the power of sleep and make it work for you.

Stop Chasing Sleep – Why Letting Go Might Help You Sleep Better

One of the most powerful shifts you can make when struggling with sleep is to simply stop trying so hard. As Heather Darwall-Smith, author of How to Be Awake (So You Can Sleep Through the Night), explains the more we focus on needing to sleep, the more pressure we put on ourselves and the harder it becomes.

Think of sleep like a butterfly, the more you chase it, the more it flutters out of reach. But when you sit still, gently and calmly, it's more likely to come and settle.

So rather than lying in bed stressing about how exhausted you'll feel tomorrow, try focusing on rest instead. Let your body relax, breathe deeply and take the pressure off. Sleep is more likely to follow when you stop trying to force it.

"Sometimes, the obsession with perfect sleep hygiene is what's keeping us up. The pressure to do everything 'right' creates anxiety that sabotages sleep."

The Hormone-sleep Connection -
Why Sleep Disruptions Happen

Before we start talking about strategies to improve sleep during menopause, let's look at how hormonal changes during this stage of life can significantly impact the quality of your sleep.

It starts with oestrogen and progesterone. These hormones play a key role in regulating neurotransmitters that control the sleep-wake cycle. When oestrogen levels decline, it disrupts thermoregulation, the body's ability to manage temperature, causing night sweats that can wake you up repeatedly. Oestrogen also helps maintain serotonin levels, which are vital for producing melatonin, the 'sleep hormone.' Lower oestrogen can reduce melatonin production, making it harder to fall and stay asleep.

Progesterone, often called the 'calming hormone', supports relaxation and breathing during sleep. A decline in progesterone can lead to issues like disrupted breathing or even sleep apnoea, which interrupts the natural sleep cycle.

But it's not just these two hormones. Melatonin, which naturally decreases with age, drops even further during menopause, which makes it even more challenging to maintain deep, restful sleep.

"If you want to feel better, start with sleep. It's the foundation of everything, your mood, your energy and even your waistline."

Alison Bladh

Cortisol, the stress hormone, also plays a role. Cortisol levels should naturally decrease at night to allow your body to relax and prepare for sleep. However, during menopause, chronic stress and hormonal imbalances can lead to elevated cortisol levels at bedtime, making it difficult to wind down.

Finally, research shows that women with low oestrogen levels often experience less deep sleep, the restorative stage that leaves you feeling refreshed. This means even if you clock up eight hours in bed, you might still wake up feeling drained and unrested.

There's a big difference between an occasional sleepless night and the ongoing sleep disruptions or insomnia that so many women experience during menopause. Understanding the role of these hormones can help you better address the underlying causes of poor sleep.

Now, let's explore what you can do to restore balance and improve your sleep.

"It is estimated that sleep disturbances affect 40-69% of women across the menopause transition."

Understanding Sleep Struggles vs. Insomnia

The difference between occasional sleeplessness and insomnia lies in how long it lasts and the effect it has on your life.

Occasional sleep issues are often temporary, triggered by stress, a change in routine, or even lifestyle factors and they usually resolve on their own with minor adjustments.

Insomnia, however, is a more persistent condition. It's characterised by difficulty falling asleep, staying asleep, or waking too early at least three times a week for three months or more. This isn't just frustrating; it can lead to overwhelming daytime fatigue and significantly affect your ability to function in daily life.

Chronic insomnia goes even deeper, often linked to underlying health conditions, medications, or mental health challenges. Knowing the difference between these issues is key to understanding your sleep struggles and finding the right solutions to restore restful sleep.

"Dr. Patrick Flynn, known for his work in hormonal health, suggests that going to bed around 9:00 p.m. helps the body optimise hormone production during the night, especially for hormones produced by the adrenal and thyroid glands."

Key hormones affecting your sleep

Oestrogen: Helps maintain sleep by keeping body temperature stable. Low oestrogen can cause night sweats and hot flushes.

Progesterone: Known as a 'natural sleep aid' lower levels can lead to more restless nights.

Melatonin: Regulates sleep-wake cycles. It decreases with age, which can make falling asleep harder.

Cortisol: The stress hormone. High levels at night can disrupt sleep and prevent deep rest.

Serotonin: A neurotransmitter influenced by oestrogen; serotonin is essential for producing melatonin. Low oestrogen levels can reduce serotonin, impacting mood and sleep quality.

When it comes to sleep and hormone balance, Dr. Patrick Flynn's perspective offers an interesting strategy that many women could try to improve their energy and overall hormonal health. Flynn suggests that going to bed around 9:00 p.m. can make a significant difference in how well your body replenishes its hormone reserves during the night. This early bedtime allows your body to produce and store key hormones like those from the thyroid and adrenal glands more efficiently, setting you up for a better day ahead.

Flynn explains that hormones such as cortisol peak between 6:00 a.m. and 8:00 a.m., so aligning your sleep with this natural rhythm by going to bed early helps optimise hormone function. If you tend to go to bed later, even if you're sleeping for 8 or more hours, your body may not be able to restore its hormone balance as effectively.

If you're feeling drained, moody, or out of sync, consider experimenting with this earlier bedtime to see how it affects your energy and mood. It may feel like a small change, but it could be the key to helping your body regulate hormones more effectively, giving you the strength and clarity to face your day with more balance. Try it for a few weeks and notice how you feel!

Insomnia is a serious concern, affecting approximately 30% of adults each year. Notably, women are more susceptible to insomnia than men, with studies indicating that up to 60% of women experience sleep disturbances during menopause. These sleep issues are often attributed to hormonal fluctuations, stress and various lifestyle factors, making them a significant challenge for many women in this life stage.

Creating a Sleep-Inducing Environment and Relaxation Technique

When it comes to sleep, I'm sure you've heard many suggestions on how to improve the sleep hours you get, or should I say the amount of quality sleep you get. We busy women are constantly running around, multitasking between family, career and potentially caring for elderly parents. It can take a real toll on our health and well-being if we are not getting enough shut eye. What I say to my clients and what I found has worked for me to improve sleep quality is as follows: The first thing is you have to be honest with yourself. What are some of the things you are doing throughout the day and the evening that could be affecting your sleep. Write them down and then come up with a plan of what you can realistically do to improve or change some of your behaviours that are sleep stealers.

Interestingly, studies show that Glyphosate, a commonly used herbicide, has been found in various non-organic foods and could impact our body's melatonin levels, potentially affecting sleep quality. Glyphosate can interfere with pathways critical for melatonin production, indirectly lowering the levels of this vital sleep hormone. This effect can make it more difficult to fall asleep and stay asleep.

Did You Know That Your Brain Literally Washes Itself While You Sleep?

While you're sleeping, your brain literally washes itself, flushing out toxins, waste proteins and inflammatory compounds. This night-time "clean-up crew" is called the glymphatic system, and it only works during deep sleep. If you're waking up through the night or not reaching those deeper stages of rest, your brain may not have enough time to detox properly which could affect your memory, mood and even long-term brain health.

Choosing organic options where possible can help minimise glyphosate exposure, thereby supporting better melatonin levels and enhancing your sleep quality. If buying everything organic isn't an option, as it can be hard to find and pricey, focus on the Dirty Dozen a list of fruits and vegetables most likely to contain pesticide residues even after washing. These are the ones to buy organic when you can. On the other hand, the Clean Fifteen includes produce with the lowest pesticide residues, meaning they are safer to buy non-organic and can help reduce costs while still lowering exposure.

Organic food can be expensive, but even small swaps, like choosing organic for high-risk foods, can make a difference. For more information, refer to EWG's Shopper's Guide to Pesticides in Produce in the resources section at the back of this book.

Sleep Stealers: What's Getting in the Way of Your Sleep?

If you're doing all the "right things" but still waking up tired, one of these sleep stealers could be the culprit. From night sweats to late-night scrolling, here are the common disruptors that could be keeping you from sleeping well.

Night Sweats – Sudden heat surges that wake you up drenched, often due to lower oestrogen levels.

Anxiety and Worry – Hormonal shifts can heighten anxiety, causing racing thoughts that keep you awake.

Overstimulation Before Bed – Digital burnout! Scrolling through your phone, watching TV, or working late on your devices can overstimulate your brain and make it harder to wind down.

Alcohol and Caffeine – Even small amounts of caffeine and alcohol can interfere with your sleep cycle, making it harder to fall or stay asleep. (Caffeine is also found in dark chocolate!)

Room Temperature – A bedroom that's too warm or stuffy can worsen night sweats and make sleep uncomfortable.

Snoring Partner! – Disrupted sleep from a snoring partner can leave you exhausted, even after a full night in bed.

Irregular Sleep Schedule – Going to bed and waking up at different times every day confuses your body's internal clock, making it harder to settle into a sleep routine.

Stress and High Cortisol Levels – Chronic stress increases cortisol, the stress hormone, which keeps you wired and makes restful sleep difficult.

Lack of a Nighttime Wind-Down Routine – Without a calming evening ritual, your body doesn't get the signal that it's time to sleep.

Not Enough Daylight Exposure – Natural light helps regulate your circadian rhythm. Without it, your sleep-wake cycle can become disrupted.

Eating a Big Meal Close to Bed – A heavy meal too late in the evening can cause indigestion, bloating, and discomfort, making it difficult to sleep peacefully.

Restless Legs and Low Magnesium Levels – Magnesium plays a key role in muscle relaxation and sleep. A deficiency can lead to restless legs, muscle cramps, and difficulty winding down at night.

EMF Exposure (Electromagnetic Fields) – Devices like Wi-Fi routers, mobile phones, and smart devices emit electromagnetic frequencies that some research suggests may interfere with melatonin production and sleep patterns.

Blood Sugar Spikes and Drops – If your blood sugar fluctuates too much, you might wake up in the middle of the night feeling shaky, hungry, or anxious. Eating balanced meals with protein, fibre and healthy fats can help stabilise levels.

Too Much or Too Little Exercise – Regular movement can help with sleep, but intense exercise too close to bedtime can elevate cortisol, making it harder to relax.

Menopause-Related Bladder Sensitivity – Reduced oestrogen levels can lead to increased trips to the bathroom at night, disrupting deep sleep.

High Histamine Levels – Histamine isn't just responsible for allergies, it's also a neurotransmitter that plays a role in wakefulness. Some women become more sensitive to histamine-rich foods (aged cheeses, wine, fermented foods) during menopause, making them feel wired at night.

Itchy Skin – Lower oestrogen levels can reduce collagen and skin hydration, leading to dry, itchy skin that makes it uncomfortable to relax and fall asleep. Keeping skin well-moisturised and choosing breathable fabrics for sleepwear can help.

Real-Life Solutions for Restful Sleep

So now that we've looked at the most common sleep disruptors, let's shift to what *you* can do about them.

I'm all about sharing simple, practical steps that actually work in your busy life. I'm not promising you'll suddenly sleep like a baby every night but making small, manageable changes can genuinely help you sleep better and feel more rested.

For some women, HRT can be a helpful option to ease menopausal sleep disturbances, and it's worth discussing with your healthcare provider if it feels right for you. But for those of us who can't or choose not to take HRT, there are still so many lifestyle tweaks and natural tools to try.

Let's look at what's possible…

Grounding Sheets

Have you heard of grounding or earthing? I know it might sound a bit woo woo but stay with me. Grounding sheets are designed to 'ground' your body by connecting it to the earth's natural electrical charge. This is said to help reduce inflammation, improve sleep quality and even minimise night sweats and hot flushes. While there isn't solid scientific evidence to back this, many of my clients swear by them. If you're curious, it could be worth trying one to see if it helps you sleep better.

Use a Light Therapy Lamp

A few years ago, I started using a light therapy lamp after learning about its benefits for sleep. Spending 20 minutes every morning in front of it helped me sleep more soundly and wake up less during the night. Even my sceptical husband noticed an improvement in his energy levels when he gave it a try. These lamps are particularly useful during darker months and are often recommended for people with Seasonal Affective Disorder (SAD), as they mimic natural sunlight to help regulate your body's internal clock and improve your mood.

Move Your Body Daily

Daily movement is one of the simplest and most effective ways to improve your sleep. Aim for 30 minutes of activity, whether it's a brisk walk, yoga, or dancing around the house. Regular exercise helps you fall asleep faster and improves the quality of your sleep, making it deeper and more restorative.

Create a Comfortable Sleep Environment

Transform your bedroom into a haven of relaxation. Use breathable fabrics, moisture-wicking sleepwear and cooling pillows or blankets to manage night sweats. Weighted blankets are also worth considering. One of my girlfriends bought one and swears it's helped her sleep better. Keep your room cool, dark and quiet for the best possible sleep environment.

Minimise Exposure to Electromagnetic Fields (EMFs)

Electromagnetic fields (EMFs) from devices like phones, Wi-Fi routers, and smart gadgets may interfere with sleep by disrupting melatonin production and overstimulating the nervous system. Turn off your router at night, keep electronic devices out of the bedroom, and consider using an analogue alarm clock instead of your phone.

Plants like snake plants and peace lilies can help absorb some EMFs and improve air quality. Placing them near your router or in your bedroom can create a calmer, more restful environment.

Establish a Consistent Sleep Routine

Consistency is key. Try to wake up and go to bed at the same time every day, including weekends. This helps your body establish a natural sleep-wake rhythm. A hot bath 30 minutes before bed can also work wonders, as the natural drop in body temperature afterwards signals to your body that it's time to sleep.

Limit Stimulants

Caffeine, alcohol and heavy meals close to bedtime can interfere with your ability to sleep well. Avoid these in the evening to give yourself the best chance of a restful night. Don't forget caffeine can be sneaky, it's even found in dark chocolate.

Charge Your Phone in Another Room

Charging your phone in another room is a simple yet powerful habit for promoting restful sleep. Keeping your phone by your bed not only exposes you to electromagnetic fields (EMFs), which may disrupt sleep, but it also tempts you to scroll late into the night, exposing yourself to blue light that interferes with melatonin production.

I get my ladies on my 21-Day Body Reboot and Reset group programmes to do this after some resistance! But they are always amazed at how much it helps their sleep. By charging your phone elsewhere, you create a healthier, more restful sleep environment free from distractions and unnecessary EMF exposure.

Manage Night Sweats

Night sweats can make sleeping a challenge, but there are things you can do to ease the discomfort. Cooling pillows and blankets and breathable sleepwear are great options to help you stay comfortable during the night.

Reduce Screen Time Before Bed

This one's a biggie. Turn off your devices 1-2 hours before bed to avoid blue light exposure, which can disrupt your sleep. If you need to use devices, consider blue light blocking glasses to reduce the impact. Turn it off and leave it in another room to give yourself a proper screen-free wind-down.

Get More Daylight in the Morning

Natural daylight in the morning is a simple but powerful way to regulate your sleep-wake cycle. Try to get outside or sit by a window in the morning. This helps your body know when it's time to wake up and when it's time to wind down, preventing disruptions to your internal clock.

Dealing with a Snoring Partner

Sharing a bed with a snoring partner can feel like sleeping next to a chainsaw, I get it. My dear husband's snoring has certainly tested my patience! Hormonal changes can make us less tolerant of these noises, which doesn't help. Encourage your partner to try side sleeping or nasal strips and invest in some good earplugs for yourself. With a bit of patience, you'll find a way to make it work for both of you.

By trying these strategies, you can make small but meaningful changes to your sleep quality, even during menopause. Remember, it's about progress, not perfection. Start where you are and focus on what works best for you.

A calming nighttime routine can make a real difference to your sleep and routines work because they signal to your body and mind that it's time to wind down. Establishing even a small habit before bed can help create a sense of calm and prepare you for sleep. Life gets busy and we don't always get it right, but it's about starting small and building from there. For example, you could spend 20 minutes in the evening without devices or watching TV or simply read a book for 10 minutes to help your mind relax. Small steps like these can set the foundation for a better night's sleep.

Here's what my routine looks like on most evenings. I love going to bed early, so I try to wind down by 8:30 pm, starting with turning off my devices. I know this can feel challenging (because they are addictive!) but it makes such a difference. I like to make myself a chamomile or lavender tea.

On most nights, I'll have a shower and at least twice a week, I make time for a relaxing bath with Epsom salts, which really helps me unwind. Then I do my evening skincare routine, which is one of my favourite rituals. As a beauty therapist, it's my way of signalling the end of the day.

Once I'm in bed, I love to read. I usually manage around 30 minutes or until my eyes start to close on their own. Finally, I take magnesium glycinate, one of my go-to minerals for supporting sleep, it's an important part of my menopause toolkit.

This routine isn't about perfection but creating moments that help me feel relaxed and ready for sleep. Even starting with just one small habit, like reading for 10 minutes, can make a big difference over time.

Here are 4 "Sleepy Teas" perfect for winding down:

1. **Chamomile** - A classic choice for calming the mind and reducing anxiety.

2. **Lavender** - Known for its soothing aroma that eases stress and promotes relaxation.

3. **Valerian Root** - Helps reduce the time it takes to fall asleep, a natural sedative.

4. **Passionflower** – Increases relaxation by boosting GABA (Gamma-Aminobutyric Acid) levels, a neurotransmitter that calms the mind and promotes restful sleep.

Sleep and Your Skin – Beauty and Wellness Strategies for Better Sleep

Menopause and lack of sleep can play havoc with your skin! There are a lot of changes happening to our skin as we transition through perimenopause and menopause, which we will talk about in chapter 10. I have worked in women's health for over 30 years and working as a beauty therapist, I have seen first-hand how lack of sleep really has a huge effect on our skin. I know in the grand scheme of things your skin may not be your first worry if you have many other menopausal symptoms to deal with, but how we look and how we feel about our appearance really does affect our confidence and happiness.

Sleep is the secret elixir for our skin that we often overlook. When you sleep your skin goes into repair mode, recovering from the day's stressors, whether that's UV rays, pollution, the environment you live and work in, or the natural ageing process. All these factors have an impact on our skin and sleep gives our skin a chance to repair and rejuvenate. Lack of sleep during menopause can give us dark circles and puffiness under our eyes, dull skin and an increase in fine lines and wrinkles. You can look in the mirror in the morning and find yourself saying "what happened?!"

When we sleep deeply, our bodies produce growth hormone, which helps repair damaged cells and boosts collagen production. This means fewer wrinkles, better skin elasticity and a healthy glow. On the other hand, a restless night can lead to more cortisol, the stress hormone, which breaks down collagen and leads to inflammation, leaving you with tired, saggy skin. Sleep is like the ultimate beauty treatment, repairing and revitalising your skin as you sleep, so you wake up looking your best! Let's look at some simple wellness strategies you can weave into your evenings. These tips are designed to help you wind down, promote restful sleep and give your skin the care it deserves. Here's how you can create a soothing and beneficial evening routine.

Temple Massage Before Bed

Massage a few drops of a pre-blended lavender or chamomile oil onto your temples before bed. Pure essential oils are too strong on their own, so choose a ready-made blend or dilute with a carrier oil like almond, jojoba, or grapeseed oil. This simple step nourishes your skin and promotes relaxation for a restful sleep.

Epsom Salt Bath

An Epsom salt bath is one of my favourite things to do in the evening: Epsom salts are high in magnesium sulfate, which the skin can absorb and have a relaxing effect on the body and is good for your skin. Use two cups of Epsom salt for a standard-size bath. Pour the Epsom salt into warm running water. You can soak in an Epsom salt bath for 15–30 minutes or up to 1 hour.

Nighttime Skincare Routine with Essential Oils

Using products that contain essential oils like lavender, rose, frankincense, or neroli can help relax facial muscles, reduce tension and calm your mind. When you apply them, give yourself a quick facial massage too. The soothing fragrance aids in relaxation, while the massage stimulates circulation, giving your skin a healthy glow.

Scalp Massage

A calming scalp massage using a few drops of lavender or rose oil can promote relaxation and ease you into a restful state. This helps stimulate hair follicles, improves circulation, and reduces stress perfect for preparing your body for sleep.

Aromatherapy Foot Cream

Massaging your feet with an aromatherapy-infused foot cream (lavender, sandalwood, or chamomile) helps soothe tired feet and calm your nervous system, which is helpful for a good night's sleep. Plus, it leaves the skin on your feet soft and well-moisturised. If you are lucky, you could get your partner to do this for you.

Night Mask

Apply a hydrating and nourishing overnight face mask This can help calm the senses, while the mask hydrates and revitalises your skin overnight.

Eye Masks

Eye masks are a fantastic addition to your skincare routine, helping to block out light for better sleep while gently relaxing the eye area. Silk masks are especially kind to your skin, reducing irritation and helping to prevent fine lines. Cooling gel masks can also soothe tired, puffy eyes, making your evening ritual both calming and rejuvenating.

Hydrating Body Lotion with Calming and Relaxing Ingredients

Apply a hydrating body lotion that contains calming ingredients like essential oils lavender, ylang-ylang, or sandalwood. Massaging the lotion into your skin not only helps lock in moisture but also provides a relaxing moment for yourself before you go to bed.

Aromatherapy Pillow Mist

This is another favourite of mine. Neal's Yard has a lovely pillow mist that can really relax you with essential oils such as lavender, chamomile, or sandalwood on your pillow before sleep. It not only promotes relaxation but also gives you a spa-like feel at home. A light spray mist is enough to help you drift into a peaceful sleep while also creating a calming environment.

Silk Pillowcase for Skin and Sleep

Switch to a silk pillowcase to not only benefit your skin but also improve your overall sleep quality. Silk is gentle on your skin, reduces friction that can lead to fine lines and wrinkles and feels luxurious, which helps you feel pampered. This is perfect for encouraging a restful night's sleep. It can also help prevent hair breakage if you find your hair is dry and brittle.

"Sleep is a natural anti-ageing remedy, enhancing our physical appearance and vitality."

Aromatherapy Candles

Aromatherapy candles infused with calming scents like lavender or chamomile can help set a tranquil mood in your bedroom, promoting relaxation and easing you into a restful sleep. Always choose high-quality candles made with natural essential oils instead of synthetic fragrances, which may irritate your skin and respiratory system, particularly during menopause.

If floral isn't your thing, try vanilla, amber, or cedarwood for a warmer, more grounding scent. And of course, always practise candle safety: never leave candles unattended and make sure they're fully extinguished before falling asleep.

"Write it down, then let it go.
Midnight worries are never wise advisors."

Alison Bladh

Night Sweat Solutions: Quick Comfort Strategies

Cooling Pillow and Mattress Topper – Invest in breathable, cooling materials designed to regulate temperature and wick away moisture.

DIY Cooling Foot Soak Before Bed – Soak your feet in cool water with Epsom salts and a few drops of peppermint oil to lower body temperature before sleep.

Peppermint Mist Spray – A quick spritz of peppermint-infused water on your face, neck, and chest can create an instant cooling effect.

Chilled Weighted Blanket – Store a weighted blanket in the fridge for 30 minutes before bed to provide gentle pressure without overheating.

Switch Sleep Direction – If one end of your bed gets warmer, try sleeping with your head at the cooler end to avoid heat build-up.

Cooling Patches – Apply cooling gel patches to your wrists, neck, or the back of your knees for instant relief.

Use a Humidifier – Adding moisture to the air can prevent dryness and overheating, helping to regulate your body temperature.

Breathable Sleepwear – Choose moisture-wicking fabrics like bamboo or cotton to keep cool and comfortable throughout the night.

Cold Pack for Pulse Points – Placing a cold pack on your wrists, ankles, or behind your knees can rapidly cool your body.

Hydrate Wisely – Drink plenty of water throughout the day, but avoid large amounts right before bed to minimise nighttime wake-ups.

Room Temperature Control – Keep your bedroom cool with a fan, open window, or air conditioning set to around 18°C (65°F).

Light Bed Covers – Swap heavy duvets for lightweight, breathable blankets or layered sheets that can be adjusted as needed.

New Non-Hormonal Option for Hot Flushes
and Night Sweats

There is now a non-hormonal prescription medication called fezolinetant that has been developed specifically to help reduce hot flushes and night sweats during menopause. It works by targeting a part of the brain involved in regulating body temperature. While it's not suitable for everyone, it may be worth discussing with your healthcare provider if hot flushes are significantly affecting your sleep. As always, I recommend speaking to a qualified professional to see if it's the right option for you.

Need a natural sleep aid?

Almonds and walnuts are packed with magnesium and melatonin, perfect for promoting better sleep.

Nutrition and Sleep

When it comes to nutrition and how that affects your sleep during menopause, there are quite a few things that can help you achieve a better night's rest. What we eat throughout the day and when we eat can affect our sleep quality and quantity.

Have you ever had a heavy meal and then gone to bed feeling stuffed! The likelihood you will sleep well after doing this is quite low as eating close to bedtime can cause discomfort and indigestion and during menopause we can feel this even more due to the decline in hormones. Indigestion and acid reflux, can make it harder to fall asleep and stay asleep. It's best to have a lighter dinner and avoid heavy foods before bed. Things to think about and start being mindful of to help with our much-needed sleep are as follows:

"Caffeine and alcohol are not the friend of the menopausal woman. They can be sleep's worst enemies."

Nutritional Sleep Disruptors

Your diet can have a big impact on your sleep quality. Here are common food habits that may be sabotaging your rest, along with actionable tips to help you make better choices:

Caffeine

Caffeine, found in coffee, tea, dark chocolate and fizzy drinks, blocks adenosine, a chemical that promotes sleep. To avoid disruptions, stop consuming caffeine at least 6-8 hours before bed. If sleep is an issue, try avoiding it completely for a few weeks to see if it helps.

Alcohol

While alcohol might make you feel drowsy, it disrupts your sleep cycles, leading to less restorative rest. Limit alcohol consumption, especially in the evening, to improve your sleep quality.

Nicotine

Nicotine is a stimulant that can keep you awake and disrupt your natural sleep patterns. Avoid smoking or using nicotine-containing products.

Spicy Foods

Spicy foods can cause indigestion and raise your body temperature, making it harder to sleep comfortably. Stick to milder meals, especially in the evening.

High Sugar Foods

Sugary snacks and desserts can cause blood sugar spikes and crashes, which may wake you up during the night. Choose snacks with protein and healthy fats instead to keep your blood sugar stable.

Fatty Foods

Diets high in saturated fats may reduce REM sleep, the most restorative phase of sleep. Fatty or fried foods can also cause indigestion, so aim for lighter meals in the evening.

Large Meals Before Bed

A big meal close to bedtime can lead to discomfort and indigestion. Try to finish eating at least two to three hours before going to bed to give your body time to digest.

Processed Foods and Additives

Highly processed foods with artificial additives or preservatives can raise cortisol, the stress hormone, and cause digestive discomfort. Opt for whole, natural foods to support better sleep.

Excessive Fluid Intake

Drinking too much fluid before bed can result in frequent trips to the bathroom, interrupting your sleep. Limit fluids at least two hours before bedtime.

Raw Vegetables

While healthy, raw vegetables are high in fibre they can be hard to digest, potentially causing bloating and discomfort that may interfere with sleep. Opt for cooked vegetables in the evening to ease digestion.

Acidic Foods

Consuming acidic foods such as tomatoes, citrus fruits, onions, garlic, dark chocolate and peppermint before you go to bed can trigger reflux, leading to discomfort and disrupted sleep. It's advisable to limit these foods in the evening to promote better rest.

These minor changes to your eating habits can make a significant difference to your sleep quality over time. Start with one or two adjustments and see what works for you.

"Sleep is not a luxury; it's a necessity. It's the foundation of physical and mental well-being."

Arianna Huffington

Task

Put your phone in another room.
You may need to buy an alarm clock!

How to Eat for Better Sleep: A Guide to Restful Nights

Nutritional Elements That Promote Better Sleep

Magnesium-Rich Foods	Helps relax muscles and calm the nervous system	Examples: Almonds, spinach, pumpkin seeds, dark chocolate, avocados
Tryptophan-Containing Foods	An amino acid that helps produce serotonin, which is converted into melatonin, the sleep hormone	Examples: Turkey, chicken, oats, bananas, dairy products
Calcium-Rich Foods	Supports melatonin production and helps with sleep regulation	Examples: Yogurt, milk, cheese, leafy greens, broccoli

Vitamin B6	Helps convert tryptophan to serotonin, promoting relaxation	Examples: Chickpeas, salmon, chicken, sunflower seeds
Complex Carbohydrates	Encourage serotonin production and reduce blood sugar spikes that can disturb sleep	Examples: Sweet potatoes, quinoa, oats, whole grains
Omega-3 Fatty Acids	Promote better quality sleep by reducing inflammation and supporting brain health	Examples: Fatty fish (like salmon), chia seeds, flaxseeds, walnuts
Melatonin-Rich Foods	Contain melatonin, which helps regulate sleep cycles	Examples: Tart cherries, walnuts, grapes
Healthy Fats	Foods like avocados, olive oil, and fatty fish contain omega-3s, which help regulate serotonin and reduce inflammation, supporting better sleep quality	Examples: Avocados, olive oil, salmon

B Vitamins (Especially B3, B5, and B12)	Help produce neurotransmitters that regulate sleep	Examples: Whole grains, eggs, seeds, poultry
Kiwi	Contains antioxidants and serotonin, which can improve sleep quality.	Studies have shown that eating kiwi can improve the onset and duration of sleep
Tart Cherry Juice	Contains natural melatonin and has been linked to improved sleep duration	Suggestion: Drink a small glass in the evening, but not too close to bedtime to avoid bathroom interruptions
Almonds and Walnuts	Rich in magnesium and melatonin	These nuts help improve sleep quality
Bananas	Contain magnesium and potassium	Help relax muscles, as well as tryptophan
Warm Milk with Nutmeg	Warm milk contains tryptophan, while nutmeg has mild sedative effects	A small warm drink before bed can be comforting and sleep-inducing
Valerian Root Tea or Supplements	Known for its calming properties	Valerian root can help support sleep, especially in cases of anxiety-related insomnia.

Low Glycemic Index (GI) Foods	Eating low-GI foods helps maintain steady blood sugar levels, reducing nighttime disruptions	Examples: Lentils, quinoa, barley, non-starchy vegetables
Mineral-Rich Broths	Bone broth provides minerals like calcium, magnesium, and phosphorus	Essentials for relaxation and sleep
Protein-Rich Evening Snack	A small portion of protein may help stabilise your blood sugar levels and provide amino acids that promote sleep	Example: Greek yogurt or a slice of turkey with a handful of nuts
Calming Herbal Infusions	Infusions of herbs like lemon balm or hops can help promote relaxation and reduce anxiety, helping you fall asleep	Example: lemon balm or hops

Tips for optimising nutrition for better sleep

Evening Routine Tip: Try adding one or two of these elements to your evening routine to enhance sleep. For instance, have a small protein-rich snack or a calming tea. Take it slowly and add in things that you feel you can do and see if they make a difference. Don't try to do everything at once because you will just get overwhelmed and give up and end up not doing anything. Be mindful of timing, avoid consuming drinks like tart cherry juice or herbal teas too close to bedtime to minimise bathroom trips during the night.

Did you know that Tart Cherry Juice Contains natural melatonin and has been linked to improved sleep duration? Drink a small glass in the evening, but not too close to bedtime to avoid getting up to go to the toilet in the night.

Have you heard of something called black seed oil that has been getting more attention for its beneficial properties and can help with sleep some latest research is saying?

Recent research suggests that black seed oil (Nigella sativa) may offer benefits for improving sleep quality, particularly due to its ability to reduce stress and regulate melatonin levels. A randomised controlled trial (see references) found that black seed oil helped improve sleep latency, duration, and overall sleep quality. It also showed potential in reducing cortisol levels, which could further enhance sleep by alleviating stress. In the famous book "The Canon of Medicine," by Ibn Sina (980-1037) it refers to black seed as being able to help stimulate the body's energy and assists in recovery from fatigue or dispiritedness. To use black seed oil for sleep, it's recommended to take one teaspoon of black seed oil in warm milk about an hour before bed. Additionally, some herbalists suggest massaging the oil on the temples to promote relaxation before sleep.

Supplements to Consider for Better Sleep

- **Magnesium Glycinate** – Supports muscle relaxation, calms the nervous system and may ease restless sleep.

- **L-Theanine + GABA** – Promotes a calm, relaxed state and helps quiet a busy mind at bedtime.

- **Adaptogens like Ashwagandha or Rhodiola** – Help regulate cortisol and support better stress response for more restful sleep.

- **Tart Cherry** – A natural source of melatonin that may help improve sleep onset and quality.

- **Zinc Picolinate or Zinc Bisglycinate** – Supports melatonin production and nervous system function.

Three Quick Wins

1. Take black seed oil before bed - In warm milk or massaged into the temples – to support deeper, more restorative sleep.

2. Get morning light exposure - Just 10 minutes outside can improve sleep the following night by resetting your body clock.

3. Write it down and let it go - Clear your mind before bed by jotting down your worries. Midnight thoughts are rarely wise advisors.

7 CLEAR THE FOG - MENTAL CLARITY, FOCUS AND BRAIN HEALTH

"Your brain is not separate from your body. What you eat, how you move, how you sleep, it all shapes your brain health."

Dr. Lisa Mosconi

(Neuroscientist, author of The XX Brain)

Five Things You'll Learn in this Chapter:

- **Why hormonal changes** during menopause impact your brain function, memory and focus.

- **How key nutrients** and brain-boosting foods support cognitive clarity.

- **The role of neurotransmitters** like serotonin, dopamine, and GABA in your mood and memory.

- **Why blood sugar balance** and hydration are vital for your mental sharpness.

- **Simple lifestyle changes** and self-care practices that enhance brain health naturally.

Oestrogen is more than just a sex hormone; it plays a vital role in many functions throughout the body, especially in the brain. Oestrogen receptors are found all over the body, and when oestrogen levels drop during peri/menopause, the effects can be significant, particularly on brain health and cognition.

One of oestrogen's key roles is as a neuroprotective hormone. It helps shield the brain from oxidative stress, a process that occurs when free radicals (harmful molecules that can damage cells) outnumber antioxidants, which neutralise them. Over time, this imbalance can lead to inflammation and ageing in the brain, wearing down its health and function.

As you enter perimenopause, you might notice symptoms like brain fog, difficulty focusing and memory lapses. Perhaps you've forgotten why you walked into a room, lost your train of thought mid-sentence, or struggled to recall names that used to come easily. These moments can feel frustrating and even alarming, leading to thoughts like, "What's wrong with me? Am I developing Alzheimer's?"

It's important to know that you are not alone, and these symptoms are common during menopause. While they can feel unsettling, understanding why they happen is the first step to addressing them. Alzheimer's, sometimes referred to as "diabetes type 3" or "diabetes of the brain," highlights the connection between brain health and blood sugar regulation. Research shows that managing blood sugar levels is vital for long-term cognitive health, as diabetes significantly increases the risk of developing Alzheimer's.

I know firsthand how disorienting these changes can be. During perimenopause, I struggled with memory issues that felt deeper than simple forgetfulness. I would lose words mid-conversation or fail to recall names and the lack of focus was equally draining. Sitting down to work often felt impossible as my mind wandered, leaving me feeling overwhelmed and out of control.

Not being able to take HRT has made navigating these symptoms even more challenging for me. But here's the encouraging part: I've discovered strategies that work not just for me, but for many of my clients too. Through small, manageable changes in diet and lifestyle, it's possible to regain mental clarity and focus. Simple steps like incorporating brain-boosting foods, regular exercise and mindfulness practices have helped me feel more in control and energised.

Did you know? During menopause, the brain undergoes a transition similar to puberty, but in reverse. As oestrogen levels drop, it can affect memory, mood, and focus, leading to brain fog. While this phase can feel overwhelming, it is temporary, and there are many ways to support your brain health during this time.

This chapter will help you understand the reasons behind these changes and guide you through practical solutions to clear the fog, sharpen your focus and support long-term brain health.

Why Brain Fog and Focus Issues Happen During Menopause

Your brain needs oestrogen, progesterone and testosterone and when these hormones decline we see changes in our cognition. So why is this? The good news is that, according to the SWAN (Study of Women's Health Across the Nation), the cognitive changes during menopause don't affect our ability to learn. Research shows these changes in memory and concentration are malleable, meaning that with lifestyle adjustments like diet and mental exercises, the brain can continue to adapt and improve. So, while brain fog can feel discouraging, it doesn't limit your ability to grow and learn throughout life.

Oestrogen Decline and Cognitive Impact

Oestrogen plays a neuroprotective role, especially in areas of the brain that handle memory and mood regulation. When oestrogen levels drop during menopause, areas like the hippocampus, which is crucial for memory, are affected. This decline can lead to memory lapses and difficulty concentrating, which is why many women report 'brain fog' during menopause.

Testosterone's Role in Brain Function

As we've already discussed, testosterone isn't just a male hormone, women produce small amounts of it too and it plays a significant role in brain function. It helps maintain memory, focus and mood. When testosterone levels decline during menopause, it can lead to brain fog, a drop in motivation and difficulties with concentration. Lower testosterone can also contribute to fatigue, which only makes cognitive challenges feel even more frustrating.

Progesterone's Role

Progesterone, often referred to as the 'calming hormone', helps with sleep and relaxation. Its decline during menopause can lead to sleep disturbances like insomnia, which affects cognitive function and memory. Progesterone also has a neuroprotective role, helping to regulate neurotransmitters like Gamma-Aminobutyric Acid (GABA), which is essential for managing stress and promoting a sense of calm. Without sufficient progesterone, women may feel more anxious, irritable, or mentally fatigued, all of which impact focus and mental clarity.

"Brain fog isn't just 'losing your keys' it's the unsettling feeling of losing yourself. But menopause isn't the end of clarity; it's the beginning of understanding how to fuel your brain for focus, memory and confidence."

Alison Bladh

Neurotransmitter Function

Oestrogen plays a key role in supporting neurotransmitters like serotonin, dopamine and acetylcholine. When oestrogen levels drop during menopause, it can disrupt mood regulation, cognitive function and memory. This is why some women experience mood swings, brain fog, or bouts of forgetfulness. And yes, it might also explain those moments when the tiniest things set you off, like someone chewing too loudly. While it can feel overwhelming, understanding the reason behind these reactions can help you navigate them with a bit more patience and self-kindness. After all, it's just another part of the journey and it won't last forever!

Brain Structure Changes

Brain imaging studies have shown that certain regions of the brain shrink slightly during menopause, particularly the areas responsible for memory and processing speed. Research also indicates reduced brain metabolism, making it harder for your brain to use glucose efficiently, which can affect focus and mental clarity.

Hormonal Fluctuations and Stress Response

Cortisol, the stress hormone, often rises as oestrogen drops. High cortisol levels can impair memory and concentration, compounding the effects of reduced oestrogen. This combination can make it harder to focus, think clearly, or remember simple details.

Sleep Disruptions and Cognitive Decline

Many women experience sleep disturbances (as we talked about in chapter 6) during menopause, including insomnia or frequent waking due to night sweats. Poor sleep affects cognitive function, leaving you feeling mentally sluggish and less able to concentrate during the day.

So, let's take a look at what you can do because there's actually a lot that supports brain health during menopause. From the food you eat to your daily habits and even some simple brain-boosting self-care rituals, I'll guide you through practical ways to keep your mind sharp and clear.

"When we take care of our brains, everything else improves from our productivity to our peace of mind."

Arianna Huffington

Food Intolerances and Your Brain

Certain food intolerances, like gluten sensitivity, can contribute to brain fog, sluggish thinking and even mood swings. When your body struggles to process certain foods, it can trigger inflammation, which affects brain function and energy levels. Some women find that eliminating or reducing common triggers, such as gluten or dairy, helps improve mental clarity and focus during menopause. If you often feel foggy or fatigued after eating, it may be worth experimenting with your diet to see if certain foods are affecting your brain health.

"Menopause may bring brain fog and lapses in focus, but these changes don't define you. With the right diet and lifestyle tweaks, your brain can adapt and continue to thrive. It's all about giving your mind the support it needs to grow, even when hormones shift."

Clear the Fog: Brain-Boosting Nutrition

So, what should we eat to keep our brains happy during menopause and beyond? Some areas that we don't always think about when we think of our brain health are how stress, dehydration, poor diet, blood sugar imbalances (can cause that foggy head feeling) and even gut dysbiosis (out-of-balance gut bacteria) can influence brain health and brain function.

Be mindful of how gluten and dairy affect you. If they seem to affect your concentration or leave you feeling foggy, try cutting them out for a while and see if it makes a difference.

Let's look at nutrition.

Brain-Boosting Foods for Menopausal Women

Fatty Fish

These are rich in omega-3 fatty acids, especially DHA (docosahexaenoic acid) and EPA (eicosapentaenoic acid), which are essential for brain health. They help build brain and nerve cells, support memory, and reduce inflammation.

Where to find it: In oily fish like salmon, mackerel, sardines, and trout. If you're vegetarian, flaxseeds, chia seeds, and walnuts are good plant-based sources, though they contain ALA (a precursor to DHA and EPA). Your brain is made mostly of fat, so cutting out healthy fats isn't doing it any favours.

Protein

Protein provides amino acids essential for building neurotransmitters like serotonin and dopamine, which support mood, memory and focus. It also helps stabilise blood sugar, which is key for steady energy and brain clarity.

Where to find it: Quality protein sources include eggs, poultry, oily fish, tofu, tempeh, lentils, quinoa, Greek yoghurt, and protein powders (especially helpful if you're struggling to get enough through meals).

Leafy Greens

Loaded with antioxidants like vitamin C and E, as well as folate, leafy greens help reduce oxidative stress and support brain cell health.

Where to find it: Dark leafy greens such as spinach, kale, broccoli, and Swiss chard. Add them to salads, smoothies, or meals.

Berries

Berries are packed with flavonoids and antioxidants, which help protect the brain from oxidative stress and improve communication between brain cells. Studies suggest that they can delay brain ageing and boost memory.

Where to find it: Blueberries, strawberries, blackberries, and raspberries. Add them to your yoghurt, porridge, or snack on them fresh.

Nuts and Seeds

Nuts, especially walnuts, are a great source of omega-3s and antioxidants. They support brain health, improve cognitive function, and help fight off brain fog.

Where to find it: Walnuts, almonds, pumpkin seeds, chia seeds, and flaxseeds. Add them to salads, breakfast bowls, or as a snack.

Whole Grains

Whole grains provide a steady source of energy for the brain, as they release glucose slowly into the bloodstream, helping maintain focus and concentration.

Where to find it: Oats, quinoa, brown rice and wholegrain bread. Try incorporating them into your meals for sustained energy.

Avocados

Rich in healthy monounsaturated fats, avocados support healthy blood flow to the brain, which is essential for cognitive function and memory.

Where to find it: Avocados! Use them in salads, spreads, or smoothies.

Dark Chocolate

Dark chocolate contains flavonoids, caffeine, and antioxidants, all of which have been linked to better brain function, sharper focus, and improved mood. It also promotes healthy blood flow to the brain.

Where to find it: Choose dark chocolate with at least 70% cocoa. Some brands add a lot of sugar, so always check the label before buying!

Note: It contains caffeine, so enjoy it earlier in the day and avoid close to bedtime to protect your sleep.

Turmeric

Turmeric contains curcumin, a powerful antioxidant and anti-inflammatory compound that can cross the blood-brain barrier and boost memory, reduce depression and support the growth of new brain cells.

Where to find it: Use turmeric in cooking or enjoy it as part of a latte or smoothie.

Eggs

Eggs are a great source of choline, a nutrient linked to memory and brain function. They're also rich in B vitamins, which play a key role in maintaining brain health and slowing cognitive decline.

Where to find it: In the yolks of eggs. Incorporate eggs into breakfast or snacks for a brain boost.

Green Tea

Green tea contains caffeine and L-theanine, which help improve alertness, focus, and brain function. L-theanine promotes relaxation without the drowsiness, making it a great drink for balancing energy and calm.

Where to find it: Drink green tea as a beverage throughout the day.

B Vitamins

B vitamins, especially B6, B12 and folate, support brain health by reducing levels of homocysteine, an amino acid linked to cognitive decline. They also help produce neurotransmitters, improving mood and memory.

Where to find it: Eggs, leafy greens, fish, and whole grains are all great sources.

Phytoestrogens

Phytoestrogens are plant-based compounds that have a mild oestrogen-like effect in the body, which may help support cognitive function during menopause when natural oestrogen levels decline.

Where to find it: Found in soy products like tofu, tempeh, miso, and flaxseeds.

Amino Acids

Amino acids like tyrosine and tryptophan are essential for producing neurotransmitters such as dopamine and serotonin, which are crucial for mood regulation and cognitive health. Additionally, GABA another important neurotransmitter, helps calm the nervous system and improve focus by reducing brain activity, which can become overstimulated during peri/menopause, leading to anxiety and cognitive issues.

Where to find it: You can find these amino acids in foods such as eggs, turkey, chicken, dairy products and legumes. For GABA, some foods like fermented foods, green tea and whole grains are also helpful in supporting its production.

Rosemary

Rosemary is known to enhance memory and concentration by increasing blood flow to the brain. Its scent also improves mental clarity.

Where to find it: Use fresh rosemary in cooking or try rosemary essential oil for aromatherapy.

Mushrooms

We tend to forget about mushrooms. Lion's Mane in particular could be beneficial for your mental clarity and cognitive health, especially helpful when experiencing brain fog or forgetfulness during menopause.

Lion's Mane (Hericium erinaceus) has long been valued for its ability to support brain health. It contains compounds like hericenones and erinacines, which stimulate nerve growth factor (NGF) production. NGF is essential for maintaining and regenerating neurons and this mushroom's unique properties may help support memory, focus and overall mental clarity as we age.

One notable study from Japan showed that daily Lion's Mane supplementation significantly improved cognitive function in older adults with mild cognitive impairment over 16 weeks. Participants who consumed Lion's Mane saw improvements in memory and cognitive ability, while those on a placebo did not experience the same benefits. The cognitive boost seemed to last as long as the participants took Lion's Mane, with effects diminishing after the supplement was stopped.

In other studies, Lion's Mane has shown potential for reducing oxidative stress and inflammation, which are known to impact brain health negatively. The mushroom may also help stimulate the production of brain-derived neurotrophic factor (BDNF), which is critical for cognitive resilience and adaptability over time

Where to find it: If you are interested in trying Lion's Mane, you can find it widely available as a supplement in capsule or powder form, which you can add to drinks or smoothies. You can even find it as a tea or coffee. While it's no miracle cure, adding this 'smart mushroom' to your routine may support sharper focus and clarity through the natural ups and downs of menopause.

Hydration for a Sharper Mind: Why Your Brain Needs Water

Water might seem like a basic necessity, but when it comes to brain health, it's absolutely essential. Your brain is around 75% water and even mild dehydration can impact memory, concentration and mental clarity.

When you don't drink enough water, your brain has to work harder to complete simple tasks. Dehydration can lead to fatigue, brain fog, headaches and difficulty focusing, things that many women already struggle with during menopause. If you often feel sluggish, forgetful, or mentally drained, inadequate hydration could be a contributing factor.

Aim for at least 2 litres of water per day to keep your brain functioning at its best. If you're physically active, sweat a lot, or drink caffeine (which has a mild diuretic effect), you may need even more. Herbal teas, infused water, and water-rich foods like cucumbers and watermelon can also help with hydration.

A simple way to check your hydration levels? Look at the colour of your urine. It should be pale yellow. If it's darker, it's time to reach for a glass of water! Staying hydrated is one of the easiest and most effective ways to support your brain, boost focus and keep brain fog at bay.

Did You Know?

Alzheimer's is often referred to as "Type 3 diabetes" or "diabetes of the brain" because of the role sugar plays in its development. Research shows that people with type 2 diabetes have a significantly higher risk, up to 60% higher, of developing Alzheimer's disease. This is due to the way high blood sugar levels affect the brain, leading to inflammation and damage to brain cells, contributing to cognitive decline. Managing your blood sugar levels as you age is crucial for both brain health and reducing the risk of Alzheimer's.

Boost Your Brain: Lifestyle Fixes for Mental Clarity

Food plays a big part in how your brain functions, but we can't forget how important other lifestyle choices are and how they affect our brain fog and focus. I see so many of my clients struggling with cognitive issues and making a few tweaks to your daily lifestyle habits can make all the difference. I understand nobody is perfect and we all have to live a life we can enjoy, but when menopause creeps in, we just have to give our body and brain a little more attention. So, what lifestyle habits can we tweak?

"Surround yourself with positive people who lift you up. The energy we absorb from those around us directly affects our brain health, influencing focus and mental clarity. Positivity is contagious and being around supportive people can help reduce stress, boost mood and keep your mind sharp during challenging times."

Everyday Habits for Brain Health

Avoid Smoking and Limit Alcohol
Avoid smoking completely and drink only in moderation.

Remember, alcohol is not the friend of menopausal women and certainly not a friend of our already foggy brain.

Monitor High Blood Pressure
High blood pressure can affect cognitive function, regularly monitor it to protect your brain.

Balance Your Blood Sugar
Stable blood sugar supports steady energy and mental clarity, while blood sugar spikes and crashes can worsen brain fog, mood swings and memory issues. See Chapter 3 for tips on how to balance it.

Manage Stress

Stress is not good for our brain and makes a foggy head worse. Learning to manage stress is key not only to brain health but for our overall health and wellness during menopause. See Chapter 8 on stress management.

Exercise Your Brain

Some research suggests if we keep our brain active, as in 'brain exercise,' it can help with brain fog and focus. Things like reading, learning something new or doing a puzzle can be beneficial.

Practice Mindfulness and Meditation

Mindfulness meditation trains the brain to focus on the present moment, reducing distractions and improving attention. Research shows it can increase grey matter in areas involved in learning and memory. I know it's not for everyone, but if you can do it, it really can help with mental clarity.

Actionable Tip: Dedicate five minutes a day to mindfulness meditation. Use apps like Headspace or Calm to guide you.

Stay Socially Connected

Studies show that regular contact and conversations with friends greatly support cognitive health.

Interestingly, in the world's Blue Zones regions known for their high concentration of centenarians – one of the key factors behind their longevity is a strong sense of community. People in these areas engage in daily social interactions, fostering connection and purpose, which not only enhances their lifespan but also their health span, keeping their minds sharp and reducing the risk of cognitive decline.

Prioritise Quality Sleep

Sleep is the time when our brain gets a good detox, so look at Chapter 6 for how to improve your sleep.

Watch Your Words – Complaining

Yes, I know we all do this and complaining may seem harmless, but research shows it can actually rewire your brain over time. During menopause, with all the hormonal shifts, it's easy to feel a little less happy, moody or more irritable than you used to.

When we complain frequently, we reinforce negative thought patterns, making it harder to focus on the positive. This can increase the stress hormone cortisol, which damages the brain's memory and problem-solving areas, especially the hippocampus. Over time, this can lead to trouble with memory and focus.

The good news? Just as the brain can be wired for negativity, it can also be rewired for positivity! Simple practices like gratitude and mindfulness can help reduce stress, bringing you back to a happier, more positive mindset. While venting is natural, being mindful of how often you complain can protect your brain from unnecessary stress and keep you feeling more in balance and calm. No one wants to be around someone who moans all the time!

Client Story:
Overcoming Brain Fog in a High-Pressure Job

One of my clients (Claire), worked in a high-pressure corporate environment where she often had to give presentations to large audiences. As she entered perimenopause, she started experiencing brain fog and a lack of concentration, which really affected her confidence. One of the scariest moments for her was when she found herself forgetting simple words during a key presentation. Claire had always been sharp and articulate, so this sudden shift was deeply upsetting.

She couldn't take HRT for medical reasons, which left her feeling even more worried and unsure of how to manage these symptoms. She described feeling like her mind was letting her down which added even more stress to an already challenging job.

After working together, we implemented some key dietary changes and simple lifestyle adjustments to support her brain health. We focused on adding brain-boosting foods and improving her stress levels and sleep routine. Incorporating mindfulness practices also helped her regain focus. Slowly but surely, Claire began to feel more in control again. While the brain fog didn't disappear overnight, she started noticing improvements in her mental clarity and concentration. Now, she's able to manage her work presentations with confidence again.

Brain-Boosting Rituals to Nourish Your Mind

You've learned about the everyday habits that support brain health. Now let's take it a step further with some simple, nurturing rituals. These are little acts of self-care you can weave into your day to support focus, calm your nervous system and clear the mental fog that so often comes with menopause. Try them at home, during a break, or whenever you need to reset.

1. Peppermint & Eucalyptus Essential Oil Quick Pick-Me-Up

Why it works: The scent of peppermint increases alertness and concentration, while eucalyptus helps clear the mind and enhance oxygen flow to the brain.

How to do it: Keep a small bottle of peppermint or eucalyptus essential oil at your desk. When brain fog sets in, place a drop on your wrist or a tissue, inhale deeply, and enjoy the refreshing scent.

Benefit: Instantly invigorates your senses, sharpens focus, and helps combat mental sluggishness.

2. Hydration Ritual with Electrolytes

Why it works: Dehydration can worsen brain fog and reduce focus, while electrolytes help maintain fluid balance and support brain function.

How to do it: Start your day with a glass of water mixed with electrolytes to rehydrate effectively.

Benefit: Boosts hydration, improves cognitive clarity, and helps you feel more focused.

3. Scalp Massage for Relaxation and Focus

Why it works: Increases circulation to the brain, reduces stress and promotes relaxation.

How to do it: Use your fingertips to massage your scalp in circular motions for a few minutes. For added benefits, incorporate lavender or rosemary essential oil. Alternatively, something I love as it feels so good on the scalp is a Gua Sha comb - a smooth, flat comb-like tool traditionally used in Chinese medicine - to massage and stimulate the scalp, promoting better circulation and relieving tension.

Benefit: Enhances mental clarity, reduces stress, and leaves you feeling refreshed and focused.

4. Aromatherapy for Mental Clarity

Why it works: Essential oils like rosemary, lemon and eucalyptus are known to enhance cognitive function.

How to do it: Use a diffuser, oil burner, apply a small amount to your wrists, or add a few drops to a warm bath.

Benefit: Clears mental fog and enhances focus.

5. Nature Bathing Therapy

Why it works: Spending time in nature reduces stress hormones and improves cognitive function.

How to do it: Walk in a park, sit under a tree, or listen to the sounds of nature. Even opening a window to let in fresh air can help.

Benefit: Restores mental energy and boosts creativity.

6. Mindful Movement Breaks

Why it works: Gentle movement like yoga or stretching increases blood flow to the brain.

How to do it: Take a 10-minute walk, stretch at your desk, or try a short yoga flow during breaks.

Benefit: Recharges your mind and relieves mental fatigue.

7. Acupressure for Mental Energy

Why it works: Stimulating specific pressure points can improve concentration and reduce brain fog.

How to do it: Gently massage the point between your eyebrows (third eye) or the base of your thumb for a few minutes.

Benefit: Promotes focus and reduces stress.

8. Brain-Healthy Snacking

Why it works: Foods rich in antioxidants and omega-3s nourish the brain.

How to do it: Keep snacks like walnuts, blueberries, or dark chocolate (low sugar) nearby for a quick energy boost.

Benefit: Supports cognitive function and keeps your energy stable.

9. Gratitude Journaling

Why it works: Practicing gratitude shifts focus to positive thoughts, reducing mental clutter.

How to do it: Write down three things you're grateful for every evening.

Benefit: Clears your mind and enhances emotional well-being.

10. Cold Splash Reset

Why it works: Splashing cold water on your face activates the vagus nerve, which calms the nervous system.

How to do it: Gently splash cold water on your face or use a cold compress on your neck.

Benefit: Refreshes your mind and reduces anxiety.

11. Brain Dump Before Bed

Why it works: Writing down thoughts clears mental clutter, helping your brain wind down.

How to do it: Spend five minutes jotting down tasks, worries, or plans for the next day.

Benefit: Encourages peaceful, restful sleep.

12. Music for Mental Clarity

Why it works: Certain types of music, like classical or nature sounds, enhance focus.

How to do it: Create a playlist of calming or instrumental music to play during focused work sessions.

Benefit: Improves productivity and concentration.

13. Breathing Exercises

Why it works: Deep breathing calms the nervous system and improves oxygen flow to the brain.

How to do it: Try 4-7-8 breathing: inhale for 4 counts, hold for 7, exhale for 8. Repeat for 2-3 minutes.

Benefit: Reduces stress and sharpens focus.

14. Herbal Tea Ritual

Why it works: Calming herbs like ginseng or lemon balm improve brain function and reduce stress.

How to do it: Brew a cup of herbal tea mid-morning or in the afternoon. Sip slowly while focusing on the warmth and aroma.

Benefit: Enhances mental clarity and promotes calm.

15. Art or Creative Breaks

Why it works: Creative activities like drawing or journaling activate different parts of the brain, enhancing problem-solving skills.

How to do it: Take 10 minutes to doodle, colour, or write freely.

Benefit: Rejuvenates your mind and boosts creativity.

These self-care acts are easy to implement and designed to support your brain health while helping you feel good and energised. Start with one or two that resonate with you and see how they can make a difference in your mental clarity and focus.

Supplements to Consider for Mental Clarity and Brain Health

- **Omega-3 (EPA & DHA)** – Supports brain structure, memory and reduces inflammation linked to brain fog.

- **Magnesium Threonate** – Supports mental clarity and cognitive performance.

- **Lion's Mane Mushroom** – A natural nootropic that helps nerve regeneration and supports long-term brain health.

- **Activated B Complex** – Boosts brain energy, neurotransmitter function and supports oestrogen detox. Particularly important are vitamin B12 and B6, which help reduce brain inflammation, support mood regulation and improve cognitive performance.

- **Acetyl-L-Carnitine (ALCAR)** – Supports mitochondrial energy in brain cells and mental stamina.

- **Multi-Strain Probiotic** – Enhances the gut-brain connection, supports mood, focus and reduces brain inflammation.

- **Vitamin D3** – Essential for brain health, mood balance and cognitive function. Low levels are linked to memory issues and mental fatigue, especially during menopause.

Three Quick Wins

1. Change Your Route

Take a different route to work or the shops to stimulate brain pathways and encourage neuroplasticity. A change in scenery sparks new neural activity.

2. Brain Fuel Snack

Eat a small handful of walnuts or a boiled egg mid-morning. Both are rich in nutrients (like omega-3s and choline) that nourish your brain and boost memory.

3. 5-Minute Brain Recharge

Close your eyes and practise deep nasal breathing for 3–5 minutes. It increases oxygen flow to the brain, calms the nervous system, and improves focus, great for an afternoon reset.

8 STRESS LESS - CONQUERING ANXIETY AND FINDING PEACE

"Stress is the rubbish of modern life. We all generate it,
but if you don't dispose of it properly, it will pile up
and overtake your life."

Danzae Pace

Five Things You'll Learn in this Chapter:

- **How hormonal shifts during menopause impact your stress response** – and why you may be feeling more anxious, overwhelmed, or emotionally reactive than usual.

- **The real role of cortisol** – understanding how chronic stress affects your physical and mental health, and how to reduce it.

- **How nutrition directly supports your nervous system** – including what to eat (and what to avoid) to stay calm and centred.

- **How to use simple lifestyle habits and wellness** rituals – to lower your stress naturally, even on the busiest of days.

- **How to communicate your needs and experiences to others** – so you feel supported, understood, and no longer isolated during menopause.

Stress is the silent killer. It is something I see every day with my clients and how it eats away at their health and happiness. It has a negative effect on our quality of life. I often wonder what has happened in society today that almost everyone seems to be suffering from chronic stress?

When we get into our 40s and are knocking on the perimenopausal door, we often find our stress levels becoming higher and you may feel more stressed on a daily basis. As women, we are the carers looking after our families, our homes, and catering to everyone's needs. Add to that demanding careers and ageing parents who need care and it's no wonder we feel stressed and anxious! Do you ever feel you are always doing everything that everyone else wants and never what you want to do? All this combined with the hormonal changes that hit around this time can become too much, leaving us feeling like we can't cope.

Many of my clients begin to suffer from anxiety, often for the first time, feeling anxious over minor things. Stress also affects our skin and can speed up ageing, among other things. What I want to explain in this chapter is why you may be feeling more stressed or anxious and most importantly, what you can do about it without causing yourself more stress! I will share how you can manage stress daily in ways that work for you including nutritional tweaks, lifestyle changes and some of nature's stress-busting remedies.

We all know that we need to look after ourselves or at least, most of us do. The hard part isn't knowing what to do, it's actually making the time to do it. Taking action often feels like the biggest challenge. Personally, I've changed my holidays, swapping 'fly and flop' escapes for health and wellness retreats, proving to myself that intentional changes can help us not only feel better and look better but also de-stress from the demands of daily life as we age. This chapter is here to help you turn those good intentions into habits that truly make a difference.

"You don't always need a plan. Sometimes you just need to breathe, trust, let go, and see what happens."

Mandy Hale

Understanding the Impact of menopause on Stress and Anxiety

So, what's really going on as we hit menopause? The hormonal changes of perimenopause and menopause don't just affect our physical health, they can also have a significant impact on how we handle stress and anxiety. Here's a clear and easy-to-follow explanation of why you might be feeling more stressed or anxious during this phase of life.

Hormonal Changes

Oestrogen Decline

Oestrogen, often called the 'diva' of your hormones, has a soothing influence on the brain, helping to regulate mood-boosting neurotransmitters like serotonin and dopamine. When this diva fades, it can leave you feeling more anxious, irritable and sensitive to stress.

Progesterone Decline

Progesterone is your calming best friend, the one who gives you a warm hug and offers a cup of tea when things feel overwhelming, especially when the diva is throwing a tantrum. As levels decline, you might notice more restlessness, difficulty unwinding and an inability to handle stress.

Testosterone Decline

Testosterone supports motivation and focus. Its reduction during menopause can contribute to feelings of fatigue, low energy and reduced mental resilience.

Increased Cortisol

Stress Hormone Spike: Lower oestrogen can trigger an increase in cortisol, the primary stress hormone. Elevated cortisol levels make it harder to manage stress and may heighten feelings of overwhelm.

Sleep Disruptions

Night Sweats and Insomnia: Hormonal shifts can wreak havoc on sleep patterns, leaving you exhausted. Poor sleep exacerbates stress and anxiety, creating a cycle that can feel hard to break.

"Sometimes the most important thing in a whole day is the rest we take between two deep breaths."

Etty Hillesum

Brain Changes

Neuroplasticity Decline: The brain's ability to adapt and rewire slows as your hormones drop, making it harder to recover from stress or process emotions effectively.

Amygdala Sensitivity: The amygdala, the brain's emotional centre, can become more reactive during hormonal fluctuations, increasing feelings of anxiety.

Gut-Brain Connection

Gut Microbiome Shifts: Hormonal changes can alter gut bacteria, which play a key role in producing serotonin, the "feel-good" neurotransmitter. An imbalanced gut can worsen anxiety and stress.

Blood Sugar Imbalances

Impact on Mood: Menopause-related insulin sensitivity changes can lead to blood sugar spikes and crashes, triggering irritability and anxiety.

Systemic Inflammation: Chronic stress increases inflammation in the body, which can worsen menopausal symptoms like joint pain or fatigue, creating a vicious cycle of stress and discomfort.

Loss of Resilience

Physical Recovery: As we age, the body's ability to bounce back from physical and emotional stress diminishes, making everyday challenges feel more overwhelming.

Life Stressors

Juggling Responsibilities: Many women in this stage are caring for children, managing demanding careers and supporting ageing parents. Combined with hormonal shifts, it's no wonder life feels overwhelming.

Decline in Social Connection

Loneliness and Isolation: Changes in roles or relationships during menopause can lead to feelings of isolation, increasing stress and anxiety.

Dopamine and Motivation

Reduced Dopamine: Lower levels of dopamine, the neurotransmitter responsible for motivation, can make stress feel more overwhelming and affect your sense of joy or achievement.

Unresolved Emotional Trauma

Resurfacing Issues: Hormonal shifts can make past emotional traumas or unresolved issues come to the surface, increasing stress if not addressed.

Understanding these changes can help you realise that stress and anxiety during menopause aren't just "in your head" but are influenced by real physiological shifts. The good news is that you can manage these feelings with the right strategies. You're not alone in this journey and there are steps you can take to regain balance and calm.

"Stress isn't just a feeling, it's a signal. Your body is telling you that something needs to change. Listen to it, because ignoring stress today will cost you your health tomorrow."

Alison Bladh

The Stress Audit.
What are Your Stress Triggers Throughout the Day?

Before we get into the actionable part of this chapter, I want you to do a stress audit. This is what I do with my clients and it works a treat. Ask yourself this question: Has stress become your identity?

Many of us go about our daily life and don't truly understand what triggers our stress throughout the day. Until you understand what is causing the stress, it's very difficult to do anything about it. Understanding your personal triggers is the first step to managing it successfully. So let's do a stress audit. Don't worry, it's not difficult but you have to be honest when you fill it in.

"Your body is like a finely tuned machine. To keep it running smoothly, you need to fuel it properly. Eating balanced meals at the right times is key to keeping everything in check."

The Stress Audit

How to Complete the Stress Audit Form

You can fill this in directly in the book or download a printable version using the QR code below.

Life Area: This section is already filled in with key areas like work, personal relationships, health and finances. You just need to reflect on which specific areas of your life are causing stress.

Stressor (Examples): In each life area, think about specific things that are causing you stress. For example, under "Work," you might list deadlines or unsupportive colleagues. Add personal stressors relevant to your situation.

Impact Level (1-5): Rate the impact each stressor has on your life. A score of "1" would mean it's a minor stressor, while "5" means it's having a big impact on your well-being.

Possible Solutions/Actions to Reduce Stress: Think about actions you could take to reduce the stress in each area. For instance, if lack of sleep is affecting your health, you could improve your bedtime routine or reducing screen time before bed.

Example Stress Audit Form

No	Life Area	Stressor (examples)	Impact Level 1-5, (5 being highest)	Possible Solutions/ Actions to Reduce Stress
1	Work	Deadlines		
		Unsupportive colleagues		
		Inadequate resources		
2	Personal Relationships	Communication issues		
		Conflicting schedules		
3	Health	Lack of sleep		
		Dietary issues		
4	Financial	Unexpected expenses		
		Debt		
5	Environment	Noisy neighbours		
		Commute issues		
6	Personal Development	Lack of time for hobbies		
		Not progressing in		

		learning goals		
7	Other [Specific Stressor]			
	Other [Specific Stressor]			

When you have done it, reflect on how you can come up with simple practical solutions. Take your time to reflect and make changes that feel manageable. Small changes last. An example could be I don't have time to eat breakfast in the morning because I'm too busy so I grab something unhealthy on the way to work. Solution, have something in the fridge you can grab and take to work with you. Like a boiled egg and a handful of nuts. Some Greek yogurt with some nuts and seeds.

Instantly Changing Your State – A Powerful Tool for Managing Anxiety

We've talked about how menopause can heighten stress and anxiety, making even the smallest things feel overwhelming. But before we go any further, I want to give you something you can use right now a simple but powerful tool that can shift your emotional state in seconds.

I have followed Tony Robbins' work for years and one of the most valuable things I've learned from him is this: your emotions don't just happen to you, your body, your breath and your focus create them. That means if you change what you do with your body, you can instantly change how you feel.

Your State = Your Emotions + Your Physiology

Your state is your mental and physical condition in any given moment. If you're feeling anxious, exhausted, or stuck in negativity, you don't have to stay there. You have the power to interrupt that pattern and reset your emotional state, but it starts with your body.

Tony always says: **"Motion creates emotion."**

Think about it. Have you ever noticed how your body slumps when you feel low? How your breathing becomes shallow when you're anxious? How your thoughts spiral when you're stuck in stress? By shifting your body, you shift your mind.

How to Change Your State in 3 Simple Steps:

1. Change Your Physiology – Move Your Body.

Stand up, stretch, shake out your hands, do some jumping jacks, or take a quick walk. If you've been sitting hunched over, straighten your back, pull your shoulders back and take up space. When you move with energy and confidence, your brain catches up and starts producing the emotions that match.

Try this now: Stand up, take a power pose, feet shoulder-width apart, hands on hips, chest lifted and hold it for 30 seconds. Feel the shift? Your body is already sending new signals to your brain.

2. Change Your Breathing – Control Your Nervous System.

When we're stressed, we breathe shallowly, which sends a signal to our brain that we're in danger, even when we're not. The fastest way to calm anxiety is to take control of your breath.

Try this now: Inhale deeply for 4 seconds, hold your breath for 4 seconds, exhale slowly for 4 seconds, repeat for a few rounds.

This instantly resets your nervous system, lowers cortisol (your stress hormone), and helps you feel grounded.

3. Change Your Focus – Shift Your Thoughts

What you focus on, you feel. If you constantly think about how stressed and overwhelmed you are, that's exactly how you'll feel. Instead, shift your focus to something empowering.

Ask yourself: "What's one thing I can control right now? What am I grateful for in this moment? What's a small action I can take to feel better?"

By changing your body, breath and focus, you instantly take control of your emotional state instead of letting stress control you.

My Go-To State Change Trick

Whenever I feel stress creeping in, I stand up and move. Sometimes it's jumping jacks, a few squats, or a quick walk around the room. It might sound simple, but trust me, it works. Within seconds, my energy shifts and I feel in control again.

Next time you feel menopause anxiety creeping in, don't sit in it change your state. Get up, move, breathe and shift your focus. You have the power to just move your body which will make you feel better right now.

How to Incorporate Stress Management into Your Daily Life with Nutrition and Lifestyle Tips and Tricks!

Once you've completed your stress audit and identified what's causing you the most stress throughout the day, it's time to take action. Let's start with something simple and powerful: nutrition. What you eat has a direct impact on how your body handles stress and making a few smart choices can make a real difference in how calm and balanced you feel.

When stress takes over, it drains the body's nutrient reserves, pulling from essential systems to keep going. It's like borrowing from one area to pay another, you need to restore what's been lost.

Balance Stress with the Right Nutrition

What we eat plays a crucial role in how we manage stress. Here are some keyways nutrition affects our stress levels.

I have a big ask for you… cut out sugar completely for just two weeks, yes, completely! Sugar can fuel anxiety, keeping you trapped in a cycle of highs and lows. Give it a try for 14 days and notice the difference in how you feel. It's a small step with the potential for a big impact on your mental well-being!

Nutrition for stress reduction

Blood Sugar Balance: Stable blood sugar prevents mood swings and fatigue. Eating whole grains, lean proteins and healthy fats keeps your energy steady.	Example: Avoid processed foods. Swap sugary snacks for nuts and seeds to maintain stable energy throughout the day.
Gut Health: A healthy gut supports a calm mind. Fermented foods with probiotics, like yoghurt or kefir, can improve digestion and reduce stress.	Example: Include probiotic-rich yoghurt in your diet to support both gut and mental health.
Omega-3 Fatty Acids: Found in fatty fish, omega-3s reduce anxiety and inflammation.	Example: Try adding salmon or chia seeds to your meals to help manage stress naturally.
Hydration: Staying hydrated helps reduce fatigue and irritability.	Example: Drink at least two litres of water daily to keep stress at bay and stay focused. If you are very active you may need more.

By focusing on whole foods, hydration and essential nutrients, you can support your body's ability to handle stress more effectively.

Simple Lifestyle Changes to Relieve Stress

Now that we've looked at how nutrition can support your stress response, let's explore the lifestyle side. What you do each day, how you move, rest and connect has a tremendous impact on how you feel. These simple yet powerful changes can help reduce stress levels, support hormone balance, and bring more calm into your life.

Embrace the power of the pause

Take intentional pauses throughout your day, even if just for a minute. Close your eyes, take a breath and remind yourself that it's okay to slow down.

Get creative

Engaging in something creative, like drawing, gardening, or writing can be a great stress reliever. It shifts your focus and allows your mind to relax.

Discover the joy of rituals

Create daily rituals, like lighting a candle and journaling in the evening, or starting your day with a few moments of stretching. These small acts can bring a sense of calm and control.

Try grounding yourself

If you're feeling overwhelmed, stand barefoot on grass or soil. It's a simple way to connect with nature and ease stress something I personally swear by.

Laugh more often

Don't underestimate the power of laughter. Watch something funny, chat with a friend who always makes you smile, or just let yourself be silly, it works wonders for stress.

Play with contrasts

Combine relaxation with a little adventure. A session in a sauna followed by a cold plunge, or even just alternating between a warm and cold shower, can leave you feeling both calm and energised.

Learn to say goodbye to 'should'

We carry a lot of unnecessary stress by feeling we "should" do certain things. Actively challenge these thoughts, ask yourself, "is this truly necessary, or can I let it go?"

Visualise your stress leaving your body

Close your eyes and imagine your stress as a colour or a shape. Then visualise it flowing out of your body, either through your breath or into the ground beneath you. It may sound a bit woo woo, but it can feel surprisingly freeing.

Try progressive muscle relaxation

Starting at your toes, tense and release each muscle group in your body, moving upward. This simple technique can quickly ease any tension you didn't realise you were holding.

Set boundaries and say no

This can be one of the hardest things to do but learning to protect your time and energy is essential for reducing stress.

Write a 'worry list' before bed

If your mind races at night, write down your worries in a notebook. By putting them on paper, you're telling your brain it doesn't need to keep revisiting them while you sleep.

Declutter your surroundings

A tidy, organised space can have a surprisingly positive effect on your mental state. Start small - a single drawer or desk can make a difference.

Immerse yourself in sound

Experiment with calming music, nature sounds, or even singing. Sound has a unique way of soothing the mind and body.

Create tech-free zones

Establish times or places where you completely switch off from screens, giving your brain a chance to reset and recharge.

Saunas and stress relief

I am a big fan of saunas and living in Scandinavia has really opened my eyes to the benefits of them. Saunas are a wonderful way to melt away stress (amongst other things!) and recharge both body and mind. The heat encourages the release of endorphins your body's natural stress relievers and improving circulation, helping to detox and relax tense muscles. For me, infrared saunas are a personal favourite. Unlike traditional saunas, they use gentle infrared light to penetrate deeper into the skin, providing a calming warmth that feels less intense but just as effective.

Studies also show that regular sauna use can help reduce stress levels, support relaxation and even boost mental clarity. And if you're feeling brave, why not finish with a cold plunge? I love jumping into the lake near where I live after a session. It's an invigorating way to energise yourself even if it can be a bit of a shock! If you can, aim for two saunas a week.

Natural Stress Busters:
Wellness Rituals for Lasting Calm

Doing small things when you have time at home can really help manage your stress load. It's just about taking 10 minutes for yourself to get your nervous system back into the parasympathetic state, the state where your body feels safe and calm and your cortisol levels naturally drop. It helps to make an 'appointment' with yourself and put it in your diary as 'Me-Time'.

In my work as a beauty therapist, I've seen firsthand how powerful small at-home rituals can be. It's not just about waiting for that once-a-year holiday, it's about building in daily moments of calm. Here are some of my favourite ways to unwind and recharge at home.

Epsom salt bath - Epsom salts are high in magnesium which your body absorbs through your skin. Having a bath with these salts can really help you relax and help you sleep. You can buy Epsom salts easily. I tend to buy a big bag so it lasts for ages.

To take an Epsom salt bath, follow these simple steps:

- **Water Temperature**: The water should be warm, ideally around 37–39°C (98–102°F), to relax your muscles without being too hot.

- **Amount of Epsom Salt**: Add 1-2 cups (about 250-500g) of Epsom salt to the bathwater.

- **Soaking Time**: Relax and soak for about 15-20 minutes to allow the magnesium to absorb through your skin, easing muscle tension and stress.

- **Afterwards:** Apply a hydrating body lotion, or one with AHAs (alpha hydroxy acids), to gently exfoliate and deeply moisturise your skin, leaving it soft and refreshed.

Adaptogens: Nature's Calm Supporters

Natural remedies often get overlooked, yet nature has given us an abundance of treasures to support our health. This was something my grandmother knew well. She was a remarkable woman with a knack for creating her own lotions and potions to address all kinds of ailments.

I vividly remember her making rose-hip syrup from the rose bushes in her garden; a remedy packed with vitamin C long before supplements were common. But what stands out most is her more unconventional methods. She would bury pieces of meat in the garden for a few weeks, then dig them up and use them on blemishes like skin tags or pigmentation marks, insisting it would help remove them. As unconventional as it sounds, her belief in the power of natural solutions left a lasting impression on me.

My grandmother lived to the age of 96, fit as a fiddle and full of life. I have a cherished photo of her at 92, playing golf with her bag slung over her shoulder like it was nothing. While I never got the chance to ask her about her menopause experience, as it was not openly discussed back then, her vitality and resourcefulness have always inspired me.

Some of nature's most fascinating gifts are adaptogens. These are natural substances, often found in herbs and roots, that help the body adapt to stress and maintain balance. They work by supporting the adrenal glands, which regulate cortisol, the body's primary stress hormone. By helping to balance cortisol levels, adaptogens can promote calmness, reduce anxiety and enhance overall resilience.

Just like my grandmother trusted nature to provide answers, you too can benefit from these incredible resources to support your well-being and help reduce stress.

Some well-known adaptogens include:

Ashwagandha: Known for reducing stress and anxiety and available as capsules, powders, or liquid extracts.

Rhodiola: This adaptogen combats stress while improving mental clarity and energy.

Holy Basil (Tulsi): Found in teas, capsules, or tinctures, it supports overall well-being and reduces stress-induced inflammation.

Maca: Known for balancing hormones and boosting energy, it is commonly available in powders or capsules.

Incorporating adaptogens into your wellness routine can be simple. You can take them as supplements, brew them in teas, or mix powdered forms into smoothies or meals. For example, you can add a teaspoon of maca powder to your morning smoothie for an energy boost or sip on a Holy Basil tea in the afternoon to unwind.

Safety Considerations for supplements: Always start with a low dose and consult a healthcare provider if you're taking medications or have underlying health conditions. While adaptogens are natural, they can interact with medications or affect blood sugar and blood pressure.

The Placebo Effect

The placebo effect fascinates me because it shows just how powerful belief and perception can be in shaping our well-being. In one study, participants were given placebo pills essentially "dummy" pills with no active ingredients and were told they were placebos. Even knowing this, participants still experienced a remarkable 28% drop in their stress levels.

What's the takeaway for you? It's that our mindset matters. A small shift in belief, that's believing in a new habit, routine, or even just hope that things can improve, can trigger real, measurable benefits. This highlights the incredible connection between the mind and body. Finding calm and clarity during menopause might sometimes start with simply believing in the steps you're taking toward wellness.

Aromatherapy Breathing

I'm a huge fan of aromatherapy oils and use them regularly with my clients to help them relax, de-stress and unwind. Aromatherapy breathing is a simple yet powerful way to calm your mind and reduce stress. Sit in a quiet space with a diffuser or burner or place a few drops of lavender or frankincense essential oil on a tissue or even keep the tissue in your pocket or tucked into your bra for an all-day calming effect.

How to do it:

- Find a quiet spot and sit comfortably.
- Add a few drops of essential oil to a diffuser or a tissue.
- Keep the tissue in your pocket or bra if you want to carry the scent with you.
- Close your eyes and take deep, slow breaths, inhaling the calming scent for five minutes.
- Focus on your breath and let go of any tension.

This quick and easy practice can lower cortisol levels, reduce stress and promote relaxation and it smells wonderful too!

Grounding for Stress Relief

Now I know you might think this sounds a bit woo woo (and we did talk about grounding blankets in the sleep section) but it does have an effect on reducing stress levels. Grounding is a practice where you connect with the earth's natural energy.

Grounding, or earthing, helps reduce stress and anxiety by connecting with the earth's natural energy, which can help lower cortisol levels and calm your mind. Typically, grounding involves walking barefoot outdoors, but there are options for those who don't have time or access to nature.

How to do it Outdoors:

- Find a natural outdoor area like a garden or beach.
- Remove your shoes and socks and walk barefoot for at least 10-15 minutes.
- Focus on your breath and the sensation of the earth beneath your feet. You can also sit or lie down on the grass to fully relax.

How to do it indoors

If you're stuck indoors at work or home, a grounding mat can help. Place it under your desk, allowing you to connect to the earth's energy while you work. It mimics the benefits of outdoor grounding, providing calming and stress-relieving effects during your busy day. There are even grounding blankets you can use on your bed.

Reducing Stress by Building Understanding with Loved Ones. You are not Making it up!

One major source of stress during menopause can be the feeling that you're going through it alone or that those around you don't fully understand what you're experiencing. This sense of being misunderstood can sometimes amplify stress and anxiety, especially when physical and emotional changes are affecting your daily life.

Opening up constructive conversations with family and friends about what's going on can significantly reduce this kind of relational stress. By helping loved ones understand that your symptoms are real, valid and part of a natural process, you create an environment that's more supportive and compassionate, allowing you to feel less isolated and more understood.

In this part I want to discuss practical ways to talk to family and friends about menopause. By fostering these conversations, you can build a strong support system, which helps lessen the anxiety and stress that can come from feeling misunderstood or unsupported.

It's difficult when you are not feeling your best and your friends and family just don't get it. You can sometimes feel like you are moaning all the time and not really getting any sympathy or someone that listens. Half the time people think you are making it up, even the doctor dismisses you with some antidepressants or some other medication that you didn't want. If you can't take HRT, then this can make you feel even more lost as most doctors aren't equipped and don't have time to give lifestyle or nutrition advice. What we want as women is someone to listen and understand this transition we are going through and to note that we are not making it up.

So how do you have a constructive conversation with family and friends that will allow them to understand what is happening and why you feel the way you do? Here are some suggestions I have seen work and I have used myself.

Here is an example of a conversion you could have with your partner. It's always best to choose a calm, neutral time to talk to your partner about what you're going through. Pick a moment when you're both relaxed, not too busy and open to listening. This helps ensure that your partner can fully understand what you're saying without distractions.

Here's an example of how you could start the conversation with your partner:

"I need to talk to you about something important. I've been going through some changes lately due to menopause and it's affecting me in ways I didn't expect. I've been more tired, foggy-headed and sometimes anxious and I want you to know this is because of hormone changes happening in my body. It's not something I can just control or snap out of; it's a part of what I'm going through. It would mean a lot to me if you could support me and understand that this isn't me making things up or exaggerating."

Here's an example of a conversation you could have with a friend:

Girlfriends are normally much easier to talk to as they get it and might well be feeling the same way. The support of our friends is so beneficial during this time.

"Hi, I've been going through some changes recently because of menopause and I just wanted to share it with you. I've been feeling more tired, less focused and sometimes quite irritated and moody. It's down to hormone shifts and I want you to know that it's not something I can control. I'm not overreacting or making excuses it's a real thing I'm dealing with. It would mean a lot if you could understand that sometimes I might not be myself and may need a bit of patience. Your understanding and support would make a huge difference."

This kind of conversation is honest, opens the door to understanding and helps your friend see what you're going through.

Key things to think about when talking to people about your menopause:

Pick the Right Time and Place	Choose a calm moment when both of you are relaxed and not stressed or busy. This will create the best environment for a supportive and understanding conversation.
Stay Calm and Don't Get Overly Emotional	It's natural to feel emotional but try to stay calm and collected during the conversation. This will help you explain yourself clearly and make it easier for the other person to understand what you're going through.
Give the Other Person Time to Talk and Ask Questions	Conversations work best when they're two-sided. After sharing your experience, give the other person time to ask questions or share their thoughts. This can lead to better understanding and empathy.
Be Honest About What You're Going Through	Open up about your symptoms whether it's mood swings, fatigue, or brain fog. This helps them understand that menopause

	is not something you can control but is a real physical and emotional experience. Talk about sex if you find your libido has dropped so your partner understands.
Explain the Hormonal Changes	Let them know that menopause is driven by hormonal shifts, which cause real changes in how you feel and act. You're not overreacting or making excuses; these symptoms are a natural part of this phase of life.
Ask for Patience and Understanding	Mention that sometimes you might not be yourself and that you may need more patience from them during this time. Explain that a little support and understanding can make a huge difference.
Mention HRT (if relevant)	If you are taking or cannot take HRT, explain this. You can say, "I'm exploring different ways to manage these symptoms naturally," or, "I'm taking HRT to help with these changes."
Use Specific Examples	Share examples of how

	menopause is affecting you, like feeling more tired, forgetful, or anxious. This makes your experience relatable and easier for them to understand.
Ask for Specific Support	Let them know how they can help. Whether it's offering a listening ear or being patient, giving them ways to support you will help them feel more involved.
Reassure Them You're Still 'You'	Remind them that although menopause brings changes, you're still the same person. It's a challenging time, but you're finding ways to manage it and appreciate their support.

Supplements to Consider for Stress and Anxiety

- **Magnesium (Glycinate or Threonate)** – Supports nervous system function, promotes relaxation and helps regulate cortisol levels. Ideal for tension, poor sleep and feeling wired-but-tired.

- **B Vitamins (especially B6 and B12)** – Vital for neurotransmitter production, energy metabolism and managing stress. A high-quality B-complex can help support mood and resilience.

- **Omega-3 (EPA & DHA)** – Powerful anti-inflammatory and stress-modulating benefits. Supports mood, reduces anxiety, and helps balance the body's stress response.

- **L-Theanine** – An amino acid found in green tea that promotes calm without sedation. Helpful for daytime stress or winding down in the evening.

- **Ashwagandha** – A clinically researched adaptogen shown to reduce cortisol levels and improve stress tolerance, especially during hormonal transitions.

- **Rhodiola Rosea** – Another adaptogen that supports energy, resilience and cognitive clarity under stress. Particularly useful for fatigue and emotional stress.

- **Probiotics (Multi-strain)** – Supports the gut-brain connection, which is crucial in regulating mood, managing anxiety and reducing stress-induced inflammation.

Three Quick Wins

1. The "Smile Hack" – Even if you don't feel like it, forcing a smile (even a fake one) can trick your brain into releasing dopamine and serotonin, instantly improving your mood and reducing stress.

2.   Humming to Calm Your Nervous System – Humming activates the vagus nerve, shifting your body from stress mode to relaxation mode. Try humming for 60 seconds when you feel overwhelmed, it's a simple yet powerful way to ease anxiety.

3.   The 16-Second Stress Reset – Inhale deeply for 4 seconds, hold for 4 seconds, exhale for 4 seconds, then pause for another 4 seconds before inhaling again. This quick cycle helps lower stress levels in less than a minute.

9 MOVEMENT YOUR WAY - FINDING FUN, FREEDOM AND STRENGTH IN MOTION

"Find something that makes you move with joy. If it feels like a chore, you won't stick with it. But if it makes you smile, you'll crave it."

Tracee Ellis Ross

Five Things You'll Learn in this Chapter:

- **Why movement feels different** during menopause and how hormonal changes impact your energy, strength and motivation to exercise.

- **How to adapt your movement style** to match your daily energy levels with the Red, Amber and Green Days approach.

- **The powerful benefits of movement** for mental clarity, sleep, bone health, mood, weight management and stress reduction.

- **How to make joyful movement a regular part** of your life even if you're short on time, motivation or energy.

- **Simple, real-life movement ideas** you can do at home or on the go that don't involve the gym and actually make you feel good.

We all know moving our bodies is good for us. It's no secret that exercise improves our overall health and well-being. But knowing and doing are two very different things, aren't they? Life gets busy, hectic even and the energy to prioritise movement often falls to the bottom of the list. When you factor in the changes that come with ageing and menopause, the idea of dragging yourself to the gym or powering through an early morning workout can feel completely out of reach, especially when you're already running on empty.

Exercise isn't just for the body, it's a mental boost too. Regular movement releases endorphins to lift your mood and increases blood flow to the brain, supporting memory and focus. Studies even show that staying active can help slow age-related cognitive decline.

I've always loved being active. Exercise for me is non-negotiable. As a child, I was constantly on the go, running around, climbing trees (and sometimes falling out to my poor mother's horror), galloping on horses and plunging into deep waters for a swim. But as I entered perimenopause, I started noticing subtle changes. My energy wasn't what it used to be and the strength I'd taken for granted started to fade. At first, I felt frustrated and a little lost. How could I keep moving the way I always had when my body just didn't feel the same anymore? It felt as if my muscles just run out of energy.

Rather than fighting against these changes, I decided to adapt. Instead of forcing myself into activities that no longer suited me, I started exploring new ways to move - ones that felt good for my body and where I was in life.

Why movement feels different now

As we've touched on in earlier chapters, the changes our bodies go through during menopause affect everything, including movement. You might once have dashed up the stairs or gone for a run without a second thought. Sure, you felt tired afterwards, but it was manageable. Now, it might feel like your energy has vanished without warning, leaving you wondering where it's gone and whether it's coming back.

I've been there. That quiet loss of energy can feel discouraging, but here's the thing: it's not about giving up, it's about adjusting. Movement during this time of life isn't about hitting the gym with the intensity of your 20s; it's about finding ways to move that feel joyful, manageable and sustainable.

"Exercise is really important to me, it's therapeutic. So if I'm ever feeling tense or stressed or like I'm about to have a meltdown, I'll put on my music and head to the gym or out for a long walk. It helps put everything in perspective."

Michelle Obama

To make it easier, I like to think of movement in three categories: red, amber and green days.

Movement Energy Zones

Red days

These are the days where just getting out of bed feels like a victory. For want of a better word, you feel like 'shit'! On red days, it's perfectly okay to rest. Listen to your body. Maybe a gentle stretch or a short walk is all you manage and that's fine. Honour your need to pause.

Amber days

Amber days are those in-between moments. You're not brimming with energy, but you can manage some light movement. Think about a yoga session, a leisurely walk, or even dancing around the kitchen to your favourite song. Amber days are about keeping things easy and enjoyable.

Green days

These are your go-getter days when you feel like you could conquer the world or at least get through a brisk walk, a swim, or a workout. Make the most of them, but remember it's about consistency, not perfection. Overdoing it will only make tomorrow a red day!

The key is to tune in to what your body needs each day and give yourself permission to adapt. Movement isn't about being rigid or achieving the impossible, it's about keeping it fun and reminding yourself that small steps still count. Even on red days doing some form of movement can really make you feel better.

Movement as Part of Your Menopausal Journey

In this chapter, we're not going to talk about punishing workouts or forcing yourself into a routine that leaves you feeling worse than before. Instead, I want to help you rediscover movement in a way that energises you, lifts you up and supports your body through perimenopause, menopause and beyond. Movement is not just about weight or fitness. It's about feeling alive, strong and connected to yourself. It's about showing up for your long-term health, one step one stretch and one movement at a time.

Let's explore how to make movement a part of your life that feels as natural and fulfilling as it did when you were a kid climbing trees or running wild like I did but tailored to who you are now. Because this isn't about going backward, it's about moving forward in a way that works for you.

Movement is Medicine – Why Staying Active is Vital During Menopause and as we Age

Before we get into why staying active is so important, let's take a moment to understand what's happening in your body and why finding the motivation to move might feel harder. And we can't blame it all on menopause - the ageing process is also quietly at work in the background. When we understand these shifts, it becomes easier to be kind to ourselves and approach movement with a supportive mindset. Here are some of the key reasons behind the drop in strength, energy and motivation to exercise that many women experience during menopause.

Why Energy and Motivation Levels Dip During Menopause

As hormones shift, you may notice a drop in energy, particularly when exercising. Here are the main reasons why this happens:

Oestrogen and testosterone decline

Oestrogen and testosterone both influence muscle health, energy and motivation. As oestrogen drops, muscle endurance and dopamine levels decline, affecting mood and drive. Lower testosterone further reduces muscle tone, strength and resilience, making staying active feel more challenging.

Cortisol and stress

Hormonal changes during menopause can disrupt cortisol levels, often leading to higher stress levels and poorer sleep. This cortisol imbalance drains energy and makes activity feel harder

Muscle Loss

Age-related muscle loss, known as sarcopenia, becomes more pronounced without regular strength training, reducing stamina and making exercise more challenging

Mitochondrial Function

Mitochondria produce cellular energy; they are the powerhouses of every cell. Efficiency of our power making factories decreases with age, especially with low oestrogen. This contributes to fatigue, making aerobic exercise harder and feeling tired after short bursts of exercise.

Insulin Sensitivity

Hormonal shifts affect insulin, leading to fluctuating blood sugar levels and energy dips, which can make high-intensity activities feel exhausting

Joint Pain and Stiffness

Menopause is associated with joint pain and stiffness, which can make movement uncomfortable or even painful. This can discourage you from engaging in physical activities.

Sleep Disruptions

Night sweats, insomnia and restless sleep are common during menopause, leaving you feeling too tired to exercise the next day.

Time Constraints

Midlife, and menopause often comes with added responsibilities like caring for ageing parents, supporting adult children, or juggling demanding careers. Finding time to prioritise movement can feel impossible.

Weight Gain and Body Image Concerns

Weight gain and changes in body shape during menopause can lead to feelings of self-consciousness. Some women feel uncomfortable working out in public or wearing workout clothing.

Did You Know?

Just 20 minutes of daily activity can significantly improve energy and reduce menopause symptoms over time.

Why Staying Active Matters Through Menopause and Beyond

Movement, whether you call it exercise or simply staying active, does so much more than improve fitness levels. For me, staying active is about living my life to the full for as long as I can. I want to be that old lady who is still hill walking and playing golf well into her 90s, just like my grandmother did. It is not just about longevity. It is about quality, staying strong, energetic and independent. Movement is also a key tool for managing menopause symptoms and boosting your overall sense of well-being as you age. Here is why finding ways to stay active that work for you is so essential.

Studies show that physical activity, especially outdoors, can lower cortisol levels and help improve emotional well-being, even after just 20-30 minutes of activity.

Bone Health and Strength

After menopause, the body's natural drop in oestrogen speeds up bone density loss, increasing the risk of osteoporosis. Weight-bearing exercises like strength training are vital for slowing this loss, improving bone strength and reducing the risk of fractures as we age.

Heart Health

The decline in oestrogen also affects heart health, raising the risk of cardiovascular issues. Regular cardiovascular activities such as brisk walking, cycling, running or dancing help maintain heart health by lowering blood pressure and improving cholesterol levels, both of which become more critical during and after menopause.

Mood, Mental Clarity and Focus

Movement stimulates the release of endorphins, our natural mood boosters. These happy hormones help combat menopausal symptoms like anxiety, depression and stress. Physical activity also improves blood flow to the brain, supporting mental clarity, focus and memory, all of which can feel a bit foggy during menopause.

Maintaining a Healthy Weight

Hormonal shifts during menopause make managing weight more challenging, especially around the midsection. Exercise helps balance metabolism and insulin sensitivity, stabilising blood sugar levels and preventing energy crashes, which supports healthy weight management and keeps you feeling energised.

Improved Sleep Quality

Struggling with sleep? Movement can help. Exercise promotes better sleep by reducing stress levels and regulating your body's natural rhythms, helping you wake up refreshed and ready to take on the day.

Reduced Hot Flushes and Night Sweats

Studies show that moderate physical activity reduces the frequency and intensity of hot flushes and night sweats, making life a little more manageable.

Boosting Confidence and Independence

Staying active helps maintain strength, coordination and balance, reducing the risk of falls and supporting independence as we age. Feeling physically strong can also boost your confidence, reminding you that age doesn't define your capabilities.

More Benefits Than You Think

From reducing the risk of metabolic syndrome and urinary incontinence to improving digestion and even easing headaches, the benefits of movement are endless. Your body was built to move and when you honour that need, it will repay you with better health and vitality.

Exercise isn't just about fitness; it's a form of self-care that empowers your body and mind to thrive through menopause and beyond. The best part? It doesn't have to be perfect or intense. What matters most is that it works for you. Your body will thank you for every step, stretch or lift you make.

Client story:
Sarah's journey to rediscovering movement

At 52, Sarah felt more tired than ever. Between juggling a demanding job, raising teenagers and dealing with the change's perimenopause brought to her body, exercise had fallen by the wayside. She had always been active in her younger years but now felt too drained to do much beyond her daily routine.

"I used to love running and yoga", Sarah admitted, "but now the thought of lacing up my trainers just feels exhausting." She also noticed her body changing in ways she didn't like. Her jeans didn't fit quite the same and she struggled with back pain and joint stiffness.

When Sarah started working with me, we focused on small, manageable changes. Instead of returning to intense workouts, she began with 10-minute daily walks. Gradually, she added in light strength training at home using resistance bands. She also started doing gentle yoga twice a week, which helped ease her stiffness and improve her sleep.

Within a few months, Sarah noticed a difference. Her energy levels increased, her back pain eased and her mood lifted. "I didn't think I could feel this good again," she says. "It's not about looking the same as I did in my 30s. It's about feeling strong, healthy and capable."

Sarah now incorporates movement into her daily life in ways that feel natural. She takes the stairs instead of the lift, does quick stretches while waiting for her coffee to brew and enjoys weekend hikes with her family. For Sarah, staying active has become about living well, not just exercising.

Embracing movement for joy and well-being

You may already be very active, which is great and please keep it up! But if you are not, and feel overwhelmed about where to start, try starting by shifting your mindset around exercise from thinking of it as a chore to more of an act of self-care that will give you a positive energy boost. Use the word movement instead of exercise as it sounds so much more appealing and gentler. I understand that painful knees, sore joints, or stiffness may demotivate you. In this case, the trick is to start small. Many of us approach fitness with an all-or-nothing attitude, but movement doesn't have to mean intense workouts and running marathons. It's all about finding joy in motion, whether through dancing, stretching, or simply walking outside. When we choose activities that make us feel happy and alive, movement becomes less about goals and more about connecting with ourselves.

Quick Energy Boost with Squats

Just a few squats can increase circulation and activate the large muscles in your legs, giving you a quick energy boost. Studies suggest doing bodyweight squats, even at your desk, can make you feel more alert throughout the day!

Explore for yourself different types of movement that give you joy. We are all unique and you might hate the things I love, but that's ok. We all need to find the things we enjoy doing so we will ideally do it every day. Try a variety of different exercises, maybe ones you haven't done before. You don't know what you might like until you try. I have a rule in my family we will give everything a go once just to see if we like it. If not, it's ok, as long as we have given it a go. You could test some high-intensity options and some low intensity, as it's good to have both in our exercise routine. Here are some ideas to get you going. Start small, choose one or two and aim to do them once or twice this week, then build on that.

Feel-Good Fitness: Real-Life Ways to Move Your Body

Dumbbells by the kettle

I keep a pair of dumbbells by the kettle and do a few reps while waiting for the water to boil. I'm British, so I drink a lot of tea! It's a quick and easy way to sneak in some strength training.

Dance in your living room

Put on your favourite music on and dance like nobody's watching. No structure is needed just move to the beat and enjoy the natural cardio and endorphin boost.

Nature walks with resistance

Add a weighted vest or wrist and ankle weights to your nature walks. The added resistance helps build strength while you enjoy some fresh air. I have some ankle weights I use when walking. It's so easy and really effective.

Get Off the Bus or Train Early

Step off a stop or two before your destination to get some extra steps in. It's a great way to add low-intensity cardio to your day without adding much extra time.

Never Take the Escalator - Always Use the Stairs

Opting for stairs over the escalator or lift is an excellent way to strengthen your legs and increase heart rate. Stairs build endurance and boost cardiovascular health in short bursts. I have had this rule for many years now and it really helps me get in a few extra exercise boosts daily.

Yoga or Stretching

Stretching or yoga relieves stiffness, keeps you flexible and offers a more calming and stress reducing way to stay active.

Walking meetings

If you can meet up with the person you are having a meeting with and do a talk and walk.

Swimming or water aerobics

Low-impact water workouts are easy on the joints and add natural resistance, perfect for a gentle workout.

Tai Chi or Qi Gong

These flowing, meditative movements improve balance, reduce stress and enhance mental clarity.

Pilates for core strength

Pilates build core strength and posture, providing essential support for muscle tone and joint health.

Group classes with friends

Join Zumba or weight training classes or low-impact aerobics with friends to make exercise social and fun.

Gardening and outdoor chores

If it's your thing and you enjoy growing things, gardening can be an effective workout with all the bending, digging and lifting, plus it brings a mental boost by getting you outdoors.

Cycling

Getting on your bike and just pedalling away is such a great way to boost your energy and blow away the cobwebs. You can even have an exercise bike at home and sit on it while you are watching your favourite series on TV.

Stand up when you are working

Use a standing desk or stand up while working when possible, to keep your body active and reduce sedentary time. I also like to sit on a balance ball instead of a chair when at my desk as it's great for your stomach muscles.

One-Minute Energy Boosts

March on the spot:

Lift your knees high and swing your arms for one minute.

Wall push-ups:

Stand a few feet from a wall, place your hands shoulder-width apart, and push in and out.

Jumping jacks:

Do a set of 10-15 to get your heart rate up!

Client story:

Rachel's journey back to movement

Rachel, a 48-year-old mother of two, had always enjoyed staying active but found herself stuck in a rut as she navigated the whirlwind ride of perimenopause. Juggling work and family left her with little time and as her energy levels dipped, she felt her motivation for exercise slipping away. Rachel had gained a bit of weight and missed the vitality she once felt but struggled to find the energy to change.

When she came to me, her goal was simple: to manage her weight and feel more energised. We started with some nutritional changes and just five to ten minutes a day of gentle movement, like stretching in the morning or a brisk walk around the block. These small steps didn't feel overwhelming, and they helped Rachel regain confidence in her body.

Over time, she added a few light resistance exercises and discovered how much she enjoyed moving again. Her energy levels improved, and she started feeling lighter, both physically and emotionally. Rachel's journey showed her that movement doesn't have to be intense or time-consuming to make a difference; small realistic steps really can lead to big changes.

Shifting to a Gentler Exercise Approach During Menopause

As we age, our bodies respond differently to exercise than they did in our 20s or 30s, and this becomes particularly noticeable during menopause. With hormonal changes, such as a drop in oestrogen and testosterone, our muscle mass, recovery ability and joint flexibility are all affected. This means that the high-intensity workouts we may have relied on in the past might no longer feel sustainable or beneficial.

High-intensity exercise, while still helpful in moderation, can elevate cortisol, the body's main stress hormone. Elevated cortisol can be problematic for women in menopause, often worsening fatigue, anxiety and sleep disruption. Over time, chronically high cortisol levels can impact sleep quality, making it more challenging to achieve restful, restorative sleep. By focusing on lower-intensity exercise like walking, swimming, yoga, or pilates, we can keep cortisol levels balanced, supporting a calmer state of mind and aiding better sleep.

These gentler forms of movement are easier on the joints, protecting them as cartilage resilience naturally decreases with age. Weight-bearing exercises, like brisk walking or resistance training, also support bone density, muscle tone and cardiovascular health all crucial benefits without the strain of high-intensity routines. Moderate activities help to manage weight, boost mood and improve energy levels, reducing menopause symptoms such as hot flushes.

Embracing a more balanced approach to movement helps you stay active, protect your energy and continue reaping the benefits of exercise for your health and wellbeing, now and in the years to come.

Pushing past your Comfort Zone – building strength and confidence

Fig.6 Your comfort zone

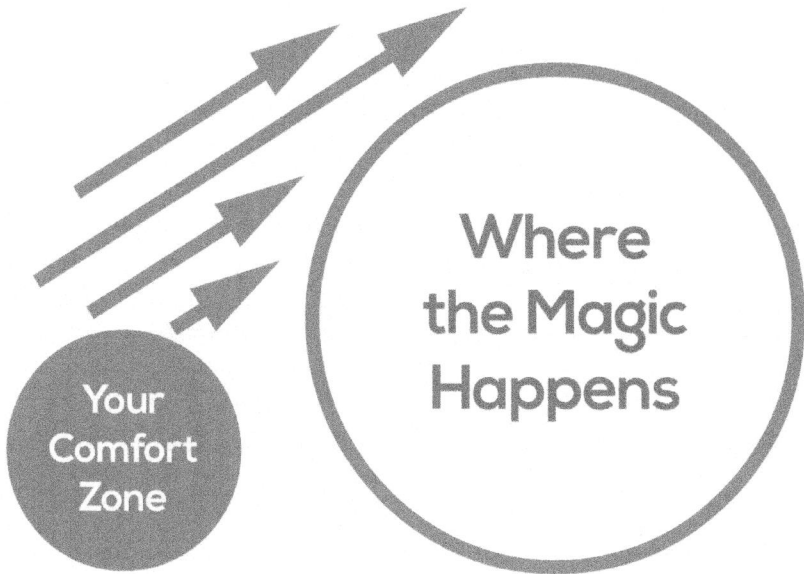

Your comfort zone is that cosy space where you feel secure and unchallenged. It's where routines feel familiar and stress stays at bay. But staying there too long can hold you back. Stepping beyond it isn't about doing something extreme, it's about gently challenging yourself to try new things.

This is especially important during menopause, a time when hormonal changes can affect your confidence. You might feel less certain about yourself or your abilities, but stepping outside your comfort zone can help rebuild that confidence.

I've always been a bit extreme when it comes to comfort zone pushes. I've done things like diving with tiger sharks or climbing Bali's highest mountain in the middle of the night. I'm not suggesting you do anything as extreme as that, but even small steps can make a big difference. Whether it's trying a new fitness class, taking up a creative hobby or exploring a new place, these minor changes can help you rediscover your resilience.

When you take small steps out of your comfort zone, you build resilience, confidence and a sense of achievement. These moments of growth remind you of your strength, both mentally and physically, helping you realise you're capable of so much more than you think.

In comfort zone	Out of comfort zone
Snuggling up on the sofa with a good book or TV program after a long day. This is cozy, predictable and no surprises.	Trying a new fitness class where you don't know anyone and you don't know the moves yet exciting but a little nerve-wracking!
Sticking to Your Regular Walking Route. You always walk the same path in your neighbourhood because it's familiar and you know exactly how long it takes.	Exploring a New Trail or Park. Trying a different route or visiting a local park you've never been to. It's a new environment that adds a bit of excitement to your routine.
Cooking Familiar Meals. You rotate the same set of recipes each week because they're easy and everyone likes them.	Experimenting with new recipes. Trying a new cuisine or ingredient. Maybe take a virtual cooking lesson or test out that new dish you've always been

	curious about.
Socialising with the same friends You catch up with your close. friends regularly and rarely meet new people.	Joining a New Social Group or Class. Attending a book club, art class, or fitness group where you can meet new people who share your interests.
Shopping at the Same shops. You always shop at familiar places for clothes, food and other needs.	Exploring local markets or boutiques. Visiting farmers' markets, craft fairs or small boutiques. It can be a fun way to find unique items and support local businesses.

As we experience the changes that come with menopause, the idea of pushing past limits can feel intimidating. Some days, even a simple walk or lifting a few weights might seem like a big ask. But stepping gently outside our comfort zones can be one of the most empowering things we do. Each small push builds not just physical strength but resilience, reminding us of what our bodies are capable of.

Many women I work with share similar stories: they want to feel strong and confident but don't want to overdo it. This lesson is about helping you find balance by taking gradual steps that push you a little further each time. You'll soon notice that even tiny, consistent challenges, whether that's an extra set of squats or an additional five minutes of walking, can bring surprising benefits, not just physically but mentally too.

Building a Balanced Routine – Flexibility, Strength and Cardiovascular Health

Example of one week's movement:

Day 1	Strength Training	Focus on simple exercises with weights or resistance bands for overall strength and tone.
Day 2	Brisk Walking or Low-Impact Cardio	Get your heart rate up with a walk in nature, a gentle dance class, or some cycling.
Day 3	Restorative Yoga or Stretching	Enjoy gentle stretches or a calming yoga flow to relax muscles and ease tension.
Day 4	Balance and Core Work	Incorporate balance exercises, such as single-leg lifts or core work, to build stability and core strength.
Day 5	Active Recovery (Light Activity)	Engage in lighter activities like a leisurely walk, gardening, or gentle swimming.
Day 6	Pilates or Core-Focused Exercise	Support core strength and posture with Pilates movements or core-focused bodyweight exercises.
Day 7	Rest Day	Allow your body and mind to fully rest, prioritising nourishment, hydration and relaxation.

The 7-Day Feel-Good Movement Challenge

Your challenge is to dedicate 10 minutes each day for the next week to intentional movement. It's not about perfection or intensity it's about discovering what feels good for your body. Here's a simple guide to help you get started:

Day 1: Walk It Out

Take a 10-15 minute walk outdoors. Breathe in fresh air and focus on how your body feels as you move.

Day 2: Stretch and Breathe

Spend 10 minutes stretching or trying a beginner yoga video. Pay attention to areas that feel tight or stiff.

Day 3: Strength snack

Grab a couple of water bottles, cans of beans or light dumbbells and do five minutes of strength exercises, like squats, wall push-ups, or bicep curls.

A strength snack is a mini strength workout you can do anytime to maintain muscle and boost metabolism. Grab water bottles, cans, or dumbbells and do 5 minutes of squats, wall push-ups, or bicep curls small moves, big benefits!

Day 4: Dance It Out

Put on your favourite high temp song and dance like no one's watching. Let go and have fun.

Day 5: Nature Bathing

If possible, head to a park or green space for a short walk or gentle movement. Bonus: Leave your phone behind to enjoy the moment.

Day 6: Balance and core focus

Try standing on one leg for 30 seconds, switching sides. Follow with a few gentle core exercises, sit-ups or seated twists.

Day 7: Active Rest

Choose a light, relaxing activity like gardening, tai chi, or simply stretching with your favourite calming playlist.

Share Your Wins

Track your progress in a journal or on your phone. There are many free apps, such as Strong, MyFitnessPal, or Nike Training Club, that can help you log workouts and stay motivated. At the end of the week, reflect on which activities you enjoyed most and how you felt after moving. The goal isn't to push hard, it's to find joy in movement and start building a habit you love.

Common Excuses with Simple Solutions

We all know movement is good for us, but that doesn't stop the excuses from creeping in. If you've ever thought "I just don't have the time" or "I'm too tired," you're not alone! Here are some of the most common barriers you can face and how to get past them.

Excuse: "I don't have time."

✓ Solution: Movement doesn't have to mean a full workout. Break it into 5-minute movement snacks throughout your day—calf raises while brushing your teeth, squats while waiting for the kettle to boil, or a quick stretch before bed. It all adds up!

Excuse: "I'm too tired."

✓ Solution: Ironically, movement gives you energy! On low-energy days (your Red Days), try a short walk, gentle yoga, or stretching instead of pushing for high-intensity workouts. Just 10 minutes of movement can refresh you rather than drain you.

Excuse: "I don't like exercise."

✓ Solution: Then don't exercise, move! Find something you enjoy, whether it's dancing in the kitchen, walking with a friend, gardening, or playing with your dog. If it makes you smile, you're more likely to stick with it.

Excuse: "I'll start next week."

✓ Solution: Start now. Even if it's just one small action: standing up and stretching, walking around the house, or doing a few squats. The hardest part is beginning, and once you do, it gets easier.
Small, realistic changes make a difference. Instead of focusing on perfection, focus on progress because some movement is always better than none!

Supplements to Consider

- **Magnesium (Citrate or Glycinate)** - Helps reduce muscle cramps, supports recovery and energy production, and promotes better sleep—especially after exercise.

- **Collagen Peptides (with Vitamin C)** - Supports joint, tendon and ligament health, helps with skin elasticity and can improve post-exercise recovery.

- **Omega-3 Fatty Acids (EPA/DHA)** - Reduce inflammation, support joint comfort and recovery, and improve cardiovascular and brain health.

- **Vitamin D3 + K2** - Essential for bone health, muscle function and calcium absorption—especially important alongside weight-bearing exercise.

- **Coenzyme Q10 (Ubiquinol)** - Boosts mitochondrial energy production, supports cardiovascular function and helps reduce exercise-related fatigue especially helpful if you're feeling low on energy.

- **B-Complex (including B12 & B6)** - Aids energy metabolism, red blood cell formation and stress resilience, all important for exercise performance and recovery.

- **Creatine Monohydrate** - Not just for athletes! Creatine helps maintain muscle mass, supports strength gains, improves exercise recovery and has growing evidence for brain health, mood and cognitive function in menopausal women.

Three Quick Wins

1. 1-Minute Wall Push-Ups –

A quick upper body strength boost you can do against any wall.

2. Ditch the Lift –

Take the stairs instead of the escalator or lift whenever you can.

3. Walk and Talk –

Take calls while walking around instead of sitting.

Please remember, the movement tips and suggestions in this chapter are intended to support your well-being and inspire you to find joy in staying active. They're not one-size-fits-all and should never replace personalised medical advice. If you have any existing health conditions, injuries or are new to exercise, it's always wise to check with your doctor or a qualified health professional before starting something new.

Listen to your body, take things at your own pace and most importantly, be kind to yourself. Movement is here to support you, not stress you.

10 BEAUTY AND SKINCARE

"Aging is out of your control. How you handle it, though,
is in your hands."

Diane Von Furstenberg

Five Things You'll Learn in this Chapter:

- How **hormonal changes** during menopause impact your skin, hair and nails.

- Why **collagen, oestrogen and testosterone** play a role in visible ageing.

- How to **build an effective skincare routine** for menopausal skin.

- The most **effective ingredients** and salon treatments for ageing skin.

- How **nutrition supports skin, hair and nail** health.

Let's be honest, when you are struggling with your health or experiencing menopause symptoms, how you look, or the state of your skin may not be priority number one. You are tired, maybe dealing with an array of different symptoms and anxiety is leaving you feeling exhausted and unhappy. Even though you may feel like you don't care about how you look, if you are really honest with yourself, you do.

We all want to feel confident and good about our appearance even in rough times. But here is the thing: how we feel about ourselves on the outside can have a huge impact on how we feel on the inside. So, it's ok to want to look your best because this will help you feel your best. Wanting to look your best does not mean you are vain. Taking a little time for self-care, salon treatments, at-home beauty rituals and skincare isn't just about vanity. It's about self-respect and nurturing yourself when you need it most. It's okay to want to look your best.

According to research 96% of women experience skin changes during menopause. 45% feel less attractive and 60% struggle to find helpful skin-care information. 80% say more needs to be done to raise awareness of the impact of menopause on skin.

"Caring for your skin isn't vanity, it's self-respect. When you feel good in your skin, you feel more confident, more vibrant, more YOU."
Alison Bladh

Having worked in the beauty industry for many years, I've seen firsthand how hormonal changes during menopause can dramatically affect our skin — not just on our faces, but across our entire bodies. As a CIDESCO-qualified beauty therapist, trained to the highest international standards, I bring both professional expertise and personal experience to this chapter. It's not just about wrinkles or fine lines, it's also about changes like sagging necks and upper arms, brown age spots on our hands, acne, pigmentation, dry or thinning hair, brittle nails, thinning eyebrows and eyelashes and even changes to your body shape. These shifts can feel overwhelming and can really knock your confidence.

I've experienced some of these struggles myself. As a teenager, I battled acne, so I know how much skin issues can affect your self-esteem and overall happiness.

In this chapter, I want to help you understand why your skin might suddenly start acting up. While hormonal decline plays a big role, we can't blame everything on menopause, the natural ageing process also has a significant impact on our skin and overall health. But the good news is, there's a lot we can do to care for our skin and beauty needs as we age.

I'll walk you through how to support your skin during this time, from understanding the changes you're experiencing to creating a skincare routine and choosing the right professional salon treatments that will work for you. I'll also share the best foods for skin health, so you can nourish your skin from the inside out. Let's focus on giving your skin the care it needs to help you feel confident and radiant at every stage of life.

"How we feel about the way we look during menopause isn't about perfection. It's about nurturing yourself, embracing the changes and feeling confident in the face you see in the mirror every day."

Understanding How Menopause Affects Your Skin

I know you are probably tired of me talking about oestrogen and progesterone (and good old testosterone!) These hormones affect our skin and we need them for many different functions, including healthy hair and nails, which can also be affected during this time.

Your Skin: More Than Just a Barrier

Your skin is your body's largest organ and during menopause, it's undergoing real and visible change. It's not just there to protect you, it helps regulate body temperature, supports immune function and responds directly to hormonal shifts. As oestrogen declines, keeping your skin healthy becomes more than just a beauty concern, it's a key part of feeling well and confident as you age.

Menopause affects more than just how a woman feels inside; it dramatically impacts her appearance, from thinning skin and saggy neck and upper arms to changes in body shape, hair, nails, eyelashes and eyebrows. Yet, no-one is talking about this.

"Your skin is a reflection of how you treat yourself. Nourish it, protect it, and wear it with confidence."

Alison Bladh

What	Fact	Why it Matters
Loss of Collagen	In the first five years after menopause, you may lose up to 30% of your skin's collagen. Collagen provides skin with strength and structure, so this decline can lead to sagging and wrinkles.	Less collagen makes the skin thinner and more prone to fine lines and wrinkles. As you approach menopause, the loss of collagen doesn't just affect your skin. It also has an impact on your hair and nails. Collagen plays a critical role in maintaining the strength and elasticity of both, so as production declines, you may notice your hair becoming thinner, more brittle, drier and prone to breakage. Similarly, your nails may grow more slowly and become more fragile, leading to splitting or breaking more easily. This is another reason that

		collagen is so important not only for maintaining glowing skin but for also supporting your nails and hair as you age.
Decreased Skin Elasticity	Oestrogen helps maintain skin elasticity. As levels drop, so does your skin's ability to "bounce back."	This can lead to looser skin, especially around the jawline and neck area.
Increased Dryness	Oestrogen also stimulates the production of sebum in the skin. Sebum is the skin's natural oil. During menopause, oil production slows down, which can lead to dry, flaky skin.	Skin may become itchy, rough in texture, or more prone to irritation/sensitivity and dehydration.
Slower Wound Healing	The skin's ability to heal itself diminishes with age and menopause further slows the process	This can make it harder for cuts, bruises, or blemishes to heal quickly.

	due to reduced blood flow and thinner skin.	
Itchy Skin (Pruritus)	Hormonal changes during menopause can make your skin feel itchy as it becomes drier and thinner. You may find yourself waking up in the middle of the night, itching like you're digging for hidden treasure! That maddening, relentless itch takes over your legs, arms, or even your back and chest and it's that kind of itch that feels like it just won't stop and you may find yourself scratching like there's no tomorrow!	Itchy skin can cause discomfort and make your skin sore and sensitive, affecting your sleep.
Increased Sensitivity	With hormonal shifts, skin becomes	You might find that products you used to

	more sensitive to irritants and allergens, often causing sensitivities, redness, rashes, or irritation.	love cause your skin to react meaning you can't use them anymore.
Hyperpigmentation and age spots	Oestrogen helps regulate melanin production. As it decreases, age spots or hyperpigmentation can become more noticeable.	Skin may develop dark patches, particularly on areas exposed to the sun.
Acne	Hormonal fluctuations during menopause can cause an increase in testosterone relative to oestrogen, triggering hormonal acne, adult-onset acne, or acne rosacea flare-ups. When I worked as a beauty therapist, I saw many women in their mid-	This type of acne can feel frustrating and unexpected, often appearing as deep, stubborn breakouts, particularly around the jawline and chin. The skin may become oilier, making it harder to manage. Understanding the hormonal connection can help you make targeted

	40s suddenly develop acne, even if they never struggled with it before.	changes to rebalance your skin and reduce flare-ups.
Increased risk of skin infections	The skin's barrier function weakens with age and hormonal changes, making it less effective at fighting off bacteria and environmental stressors.	You may notice more frequent skin infections or irritation from things like makeup or skincare products.
Changes in Skin Texture	Menopause can cause skin to become rougher, especially around areas like the elbows, knees and back of the arms.	This can leave the skin looking dull or feeling uneven to the touch.

Reduction in Subcutaneous Fat	The fat layer beneath your skin thins out during menopause, contributing to a loss of volume in the face and hands.	This can create a more hollow or sunken appearance in the cheeks and around the eyes.
Skin tags	Skin tags are small, soft, harmless growths of skin that often appear on areas where skin rubs against skin or clothing, such as the neck, armpits, under the breasts, or groin area. They are more common during menopause because of hormonal changes and slower skin cell turnover.	While they are medically harmless, skin tags can be annoying or make you feel self-conscious, especially if they appear in noticeable areas. They can also become irritated or uncomfortable when caught on clothing or jewellery.

Oestrogen Helps Maintain Skin Hydration

With declining oestrogen, the skin's ability to retain moisture decreases, often leading to dryness and sensitivity. Using moisturisers with ingredients like hyaluronic acid can help to restore hydration during menopause and beyond.

Don't Overlook Your Mucous Membranes

When talking about skin, I have to mention our mucous membranes, as these can certainly become drier during menopause and beyond. This means you need to look after your vagina. You need to give it a little more attention to keep things happy and moist down there. But dryness doesn't just affect your vagina. Your eyes, nose and mouth all have mucous membranes and can become sore and dry too.

So what are mucous membranes? They are the moist linings of areas like your eyes, nose, mouth and vagina. With the drop in oestrogen, these membranes can dry out, leading to discomfort in multiple areas of your body. You may notice dry, irritated eyes, a dry mouth, or even a stuffy nose. Vaginal dryness is also common and can make intimacy uncomfortable. Taking care of these sensitive areas is as important as looking after your skin.

So, what can we do? Staying hydrated is key. Drinking enough water throughout the day will help keep your mucous membranes moist. Humidifiers, eye drops and saline sprays can also provide relief. For vaginal dryness, non-hormonal lubricants and moisturisers are available. Additionally, if you can't or don't want to take systemic HRT but struggle with vaginal dryness, there are oestrogen creams that are applied locally and backed by research as effective non-systemic treatments. They work by relieving dryness without causing the broader hormonal effects of systemic hormone therapy. Taking care of your mucous membranes can significantly improve your overall comfort and enhance intimacy, helping you feel happier and more at ease in your body.

The vagina has its own microbiome (a community of beneficial bacteria that help maintain balance and protect against infections), similar to your gut! These "good bacteria" play a crucial role in maintaining pH balance and preventing infections. During menopause, hormonal changes can disrupt this bacterial balance, which is why extra care and hydration are key to keeping things balanced and healthy.

"Your skin tells the story of your life and how you've cared for it. Each wrinkle, line, or mark is a testament to the choices you've made along the way."

Sea Buckthorn –
A Natural Ally for Mucous Membranes

Research shows that sea buckthorn oil is rich in omega-7 fatty acids, which help nourish and protect mucous membranes throughout the body, including the eyes, mouth, and vagina. This powerful plant extract has been studied for its ability to increase hydration and support tissue health, making it a natural option for women struggling with dryness during menopause.

Adding sea buckthorn supplements to your routine may help improve vaginal comfort, relieve dry eyes and mouth and support overall skin hydration.

The Essential Skincare Routine for Menopausal Skin

So, let's talk about how to care for your skin through this stage, as it may need just a little more tender loving care (TLC). Here is an easy-to-follow skincare routine that's tailored to menopausal skin, focusing on hydration, nourishment and protection. With a little care, your skin can continue to glow with health and vitality, no matter what hormonal shifts are going on underneath.

When it comes to ingredients, here are a few of the best ones that really have an effect on the skin. It's always good to talk to a professional beauty therapist to get the correct products for your skin type. Here are some of my favourite ingredients.

Essential Skincare Ingredients for Menopausal Skin

As we age and move through menopause, our skin goes through noticeable changes. You've likely heard me say it before your skin can become drier, more sensitive, thinner and less elastic, largely due to the drop in hormones like oestrogen. But here's the good news: the right skincare ingredients can make a real difference. They can help nourish, protect and support your skin through this transition.

Below is a breakdown of the key ingredients to look for and where you'll typically find them, whether it's in your day or night cream, serums, cleansers, eye creams, neck treatments, masks or exfoliating peels.

Retinol (Vitamin A)

What it does: Retinol boosts cell turnover, reduces fine lines and stimulates collagen production, leading to firmer and more youthful-looking skin.

Types of Retinol & Retinoids in Skincare

Retinyl Palmitate → The gentlest and least potent form, ideal for beginners or sensitive skin. It takes longer to show results, as it needs to be converted into retinoic acid in the skin.

Retinol → The most commonly used form in over-the-counter skincare. It is stronger than retinyl palmitate but still requires conversion into retinoic acid to be effective. It helps with fine lines, wrinkles and uneven skin tone.

Retinaldehyde (Retinal) → A more advanced form of retinol, works faster than standard retinol but is still gentler than prescription-strength retinoids. It requires only one conversion step to become retinoic acid, making it more potent and effective for visible signs of ageing.

Retinoic Acid (Tretinoin) → The most potent form, available by prescription only (e.g., Tretinoin, Retin-A). It works immediately as it doesn't require conversion, delivering faster and more dramatic results but with a higher risk of irritation.

Retinol Esters (Retinyl Acetate, Retinyl Linoleate, Retinyl Propionate) → Milder than retinol, these esters require multiple conversion steps before becoming active, making them less irritating but slower to work.

Hyaluronic Acid

What it does: It acts as a moisture magnet, drawing water into the skin and giving it a plump, hydrated appearance, essential for dry menopausal skin.

Where to find it: Available in serums, moisturisers and hydrating masks.

AHAs (Alpha Hydroxy Acids)

What they do: AHAs such as glycolic and lactic acid gently exfoliate the skin, removing dead skin cells and revealing fresher, smoother skin underneath. They help with menopausal dryness and uneven texture.

Where to find them: Common in exfoliating cleansers, chemical peels, masks, and night creams.

Niacinamide (Vitamin B3)

What it does: Strengthens the skin barrier, reduces inflammation and helps balance oil production, which can be disrupted during menopause.

Where to find it: Often included in serums and day and night creams.

SPF 30 or Higher

What it does: Daily sun protection is crucial as skin becomes more sensitive and prone to UV damage, which accelerates ageing.

Where to find it: Look for day creams and moisturisers with at least SPF 30 to protect your skin from sun damage.

Phytoestrogens

What they do: These plant-based compounds mimic the effects of oestrogen, helping to boost skin hydration, elasticity, and firmness, key concerns for menopausal skin.

Where to find them: Typically found in day and nighttime moisturisers and serums designed for mature skin.

The skincare industry is always moving forward and when it comes to new exciting ingredients that can help our skin, here are a few emerging ingredients that have shown promise for ageing skin and have research to back them up.

Malassezin

Derived through biotechnology, malassezin is a gentler alternative to vitamin C. It offers antioxidant properties that help brighten the skin and may help reduce signs of ageing without the potential irritation associated with traditional vitamin C products. It can help reduce the appearance of dark spots, discolouration on the skin and sun damage.

Exosomes

Exosomes are tiny vesicles that facilitate cell-to-cell communication, playing a crucial role in skin regeneration and wrinkle reduction. In skincare, they help promote collagen production and improve skin elasticity, leading to a firmer and more youthful appearance.

Plant stem cells

Extracted from various plants, these stem cells are rich in antioxidants and have regenerative properties. They aid in protecting the skin from environmental damage and support the renewal of skin cells, contributing to a more radiant complexion.

Peptides

Peptides are short chains of amino acids that serve as building blocks for proteins like collagen and elastin. Incorporating peptides into skincare can stimulate collagen production, leading to firmer and smoother skin.

Sunscreen: Your Daily Non-Negotiable

If you only take one thing away from this chapter, let it be this: start using sunscreen, every single day. It's one of the most powerful tools you have to protect your skin and slow down the signs of ageing. And the earlier you start, the better.

When I was growing up in the States, the goal was to get a tan, fast. Sunscreen wasn't fashionable. If you used anything at all, it was probably SPF 2... if that! We even used mineral oil to intensify tanning. Looking back, it makes me wince. We didn't realise just how dangerous this was. The sun doesn't just give you a golden glow, it can cause serious long-term damage that builds up silently over the years. You might not notice it straight away (unless you burn, of course, which is not only painful but also increases the risk of skin cancer), but it shows up later as pigmentation, age spots, rough skin texture and premature wrinkles.

Now we know better. Research tells us we should all be using SPF 30 or higher daily. I personally use SPF 50, 365 days a year. This isn't just a summer thing. Even on cloudy days or when you're just nipping out, those UV rays are still at work.

During menopause, your skin becomes thinner, drier and more sensitive. It's also more vulnerable to UV damage, which can make all the common skin concerns worse, wrinkles, uneven tone, sagging and increased sensitivity. That's why daily sun protection isn't optional, it's essential. Think of it as one of the most important and easy steps you can take to keep your skin healthy, protected and glowing.

Did you know your skin renews itself every 28-30 days? The skin's outermost layer, the epidermis, naturally sheds and renews itself approximately every month. However, this process slows down with age, contributing to the duller complexion many women notice during and after menopause.

Most good quality day creams now contain SPF 30 or higher. Here is a list of the **SPF 30 or Higher types of sunscreens**:

Physical (Mineral) Sunscreen

Ingredients: Zinc oxide or titanium dioxide.

How it works: Sits on top of the skin and physically blocks UV rays. This type of sunscreen is great for sensitive skin as it's less likely to cause irritation.

Chemical Sunscreen

Ingredients: Oxybenzone, avobenzone, octisalate, octocrylene, homosalate and octinoxate.

How it works: Absorbs into the skin and converts UV rays into heat, which is then released from the body. Chemical sunscreens are often lighter and easier to wear daily under makeup but can sometimes irritate sensitive skin.

Broad Spectrum

This label ensures protection against both UVA (which ages the skin) and UVB (which burns the skin) rays, making it the best choice for comprehensive protection.

What to look for:

Choose sunscreens with at least SPF 30 for effective daily protection. Consider formulations with added hydrating ingredients to suit menopausal skin, which may become drier and more sensitive.

Using sunscreen daily helps maintain youthful, healthy skin and during menopause, it becomes even more critical to protect against premature ageing and other skin issues.

I always get asked about what ingredients to avoid in sunscreens, so here is a table giving you the latest information according to research.

Ingredients to avoid in sunscreens		
Ingredient	Why avoid it?	Research
Oxybenzone	Oxybenzone is a chemical UV filter that can cause skin irritation and allergies, particularly in sensitive skin. It has also been linked to hormonal disruption and may contribute to coral reef damage.	Studies suggest that oxybenzone can penetrate the skin and act as an endocrine disruptor, potentially interfering with hormone levels. Research published in Environmental Health Perspectives highlights its impact on marine ecosystems, particularly coral reefs.
Octinoxate	Octinoxate has been shown to disrupt hormones and cause allergic reactions. Like oxybenzone, it is also harmful to coral reefs.	A study in Toxicology Reports indicates that octinoxate can impact reproductive hormone levels in humans and is associated with coral bleaching in marine environments.
Homomenthyl Salicylate (Homosalate)	Homosalate is a chemical UV filter that may break down into harmful by-products over time,	The European Commission's Scientific Committee on Consumer Safety has raised concerns about homosalate's

	potentially affecting hormone regulation.	endocrine-disrupting properties and its potential to accumulate in the body.
Parabens	Parabens are preservatives that may interfere with hormone function and contribute to skin sensitivity. Manufacturers often include parabens in sunscreens to extend shelf life.	According to studies in The Journal of Applied Toxicology, parabens can mimic oestrogen in the body, potentially contributing to hormonal imbalances.
Retinyl Palmitate (Vitamin A Derivative)	While retinyl palmitate has antioxidant properties, it can break down into harmful free radicals when exposed to sunlight, potentially accelerating skin damage and increasing the risk of cancer.	A study by the National Toxicology Program found that retinyl palmitate could enhance photo carcinogenic activity, raising concerns about its inclusion in sunscreens.
Fragrance	Added fragrances in sunscreen can cause skin irritation and may	Studies published in Contact Dermatitis show that fragrances are among

	include undisclosed harmful chemicals.	the top allergens in personal care products, including sunscreens.
Nano Titanium Dioxide and Zinc Oxide	While non-nano versions of these ingredients are safe and effective, the nanoparticle forms may penetrate the skin or be inhaled, potentially causing cellular damage or respiratory issues.	Research in Nano toxicology suggests that nanoparticles could generate free radicals, which may damage skin cells or exacerbate respiratory issues if inhaled.

What to Look for Instead

Choose mineral sunscreens with non-nano zinc oxide or titanium dioxide, as these are safe, effective, and environmentally friendly. Look for broad-spectrum protection that shields against both UVA and UVB rays.

Opt for products labelled as reef-safe to ensure minimal environmental impact.

Prioritise sunscreens with added antioxidants, such as vitamin E or niacinamide, to protect against free radical damage.

By avoiding these harmful ingredients and selecting more natural, well-researched alternatives, you can protect your skin effectively.

I can't tell you how many women I've met later in life who've spent years on the golf course or out sailing with no sunscreen and their skin tells the story. But here's the good news: it's never too late to start protecting your skin and giving it the care it truly deserves.

How Screen Time is Secretly Ageing Your Skin

Our modern world and our devices can play havoc with our skin, and this is not something we think about. The good news is bio-hacking (using science-backed strategies to optimise your body and health) your skincare routine is now easier than ever with innovative creams designed to protect against blue and red light from screens. Prolonged exposure to these lights can accelerate premature ageing and weaken your skin's natural barrier. Look for products with antioxidants like vitamin C, vitamin E, or niacinamide and those labelled as "anti-blue light" or "digital defence." These creams not only neutralise free radicals but also add a layer of protection to maintain your skin's health and radiance in our screen-dominated world. If you sit in front of a computer all day, I suggest you invest in a good day cream.

Love your neck: A guide to keeping it firm!

Do you use a neck cream? Did you know the neck often reveals signs of ageing sooner than other areas? Yet it's one of the most neglected parts of skincare routines. Many of us don't apply our skincare products to the delicate neck area and certainly not on the decolletage area! Which is another issue in itself.

Studies show that only 17% of women actively care for their neck and less than a third use a neck-specific product daily. The skin on the neck is thinner, has fewer oil glands and is in constant motion, making it more vulnerable to dryness, sagging, wrinkles and pigmentation. Add in hormonal changes during menopause and the effects of 'tech neck' (those horizontal lines caused by constantly looking down at phones and screens) and these concerns can become even more noticeable.

I often get asked by women, "What can I do for my neck?" After all, no one wants a saggy neck, or what's commonly referred to as a 'turkey neck'. The good news? With a few simple steps, you can keep your neck looking firm and fabulous for years to come!

Everyday Neck Care

Caring for your neck doesn't have to be complicated. A few simple steps in your skincare routine can make a big difference:

Cleanse Gently: Use a cream cleanser daily to keep the skin clean and hydrated. Cream cleansers are best and you can use the same one you use on your face.

Hydrate and Protect: Start with a dedicated neck cream these are specially formulated to care for the thinner, more delicate skin on the neck, helping to firm, smooth and nourish. Then layer your day cream with SPF over the top to give your neck the essential sun protection it needs.

Use Targeted Treatments: Neck creams or serums containing retinol, niacinamide, or antioxidants can help stimulate collagen and improve skin texture.

Massage with Products: Use upward strokes when applying

products to boost circulation and absorption.

Adopt Healthy Habits: Maintain good posture, avoid excessive screen time, and stay hydrated to reduce strain and support skin health.

Professional Salon Treatments for the Neck

If you want more targeted results, you can always book yourself in for some salon treatments. Here are some of my favourites that can provide noticeable improvements:

Radiofrequency (RF) Skin Tightening: Stimulates collagen and elastin production to tighten sagging skin

Ultrasound Therapy (e.g., Ultherapy): Lifts and firms the deeper layers of neck skin, with results improving over months.

Microneedling with Radiofrequency: Combines microneedling and heat to reduce fine lines and improve texture.

Chemical Peels: Exfoliates the neck to smooth skin and reduce pigmentation.

Cryotherapy: Uses cold therapy to tighten the skin for a firming effect.

Laser Resurfacing: Targets wrinkles and sun damage while tightening skin and improving texture.

These treatments are tailored to the neck's delicate skin and can address specific concerns like sagging, wrinkles, or uneven tone.

By combining your daily care with occasional professional treatments, you can help to prevent turkey neck and keep your neck looking smooth, firm and youthful as you transition through menopause.

Cosmetic Procedures for Your Neck

This of course is not for everyone but it's always good to have all the options in front of you as cosmetic procedures can be an option for those wanting more advanced solutions to tackle sagging, wrinkles, or lack of definition in the neck area. Here are some popular treatments, ranging from non-invasive to surgical options:

Botox: Relaxes vertical neck bands for a smoother look.

Fillers: Softens horizontal lines and restores volume.

Skin Boosters (e.g., Profhilo): Hydrates and firms the neck, boosting collagen.

Thread Lifts: Lifts and tightens sagging skin with dissolvable threads.

Micro liposuction: Removes small fat pockets under the chin for a sleeker neck.

Kybella: Injections to dissolve fat under the chin (double chin).

Platelet-Rich Plasma (PRP) Therapy: Uses your own plasma to rejuvenate and firm the neck.

Laser Resurfacing: Improves texture and tightens the skin, targeting wrinkles and sun damage.

Surgical Options

Neck Lift: Tightens and reshapes the neck by removing excess skin and tightening muscles.

Liposuction: Removes larger fat deposits for a more defined neck and jawline.

Chin Implants: Enhances the jawline and balances proportions for a more sculpted neck.

These options cater to various needs, from subtle improvements to more dramatic results. Always speak to a qualified doctor to explore what option is best for you.

Skincare Routine

You might already have a solid routine in place and that's great! But if you're not using any products at the moment, don't worry. Let's keep it simple to begin with. Start with the basics: a gentle cleanser, a nourishing day cream, and a night cream to support your skin while you sleep. That's all you need to get going. Once you're comfortable, you can gradually add in other products like serums or eye creams when you feel ready.

Morning routine	
Cleanser	Start your morning by cleansing your skin with a gentle cream cleanser that hydrates as it works. Choose one that removes impurities without stripping away natural oils, leaving your skin soft, clean and refreshed. Cream cleansers tend to be less drying than gel-based options and are much kinder to menopausal skin, which often needs extra care and moisture.
Toner	After cleansing, use a toner to balance your skin's pH and prepare it for the rest of your skincare routine. A hydrating toner is best, particularly one that soothes and refreshes without alcohol. Many women skip this, but it is important to use a toner to rebalance the skin.
Serum	Serums are packed with active ingredients that deliver targeted results. In the morning, try a Vitamin C serum to defend your skin against free radicals and brighten your complexion. If you're looking to boost elasticity and tone, a firming peptide serum is another great option, it can help support collagen production and give your skin a smoother, lifted look as you go about your day.
Day cream with SPF 30 or higher	Moisturise and protect your skin from the sun with a day cream that includes at least SPF 30 even better if you can use 50. This is CRUCIAL for menopausal skin, which can be more prone to UV damage and sensitivity.

Neck Cream	If you want to go the extra mile, apply a neck cream to help firm and nourish this often-neglected area. If not, just remember to take your serum and day cream down to your neck and décolletage, no one wants a dry, wrinkly décolletage!

Evening routine

Eye Makeup Remover	Start your evening routine by removing eye makeup with a gentle makeup remover to avoid irritation. Using your cleanser around the eye area will cause puffiness and irritate the eyes.
Cleanser	Cleanse your face with the same hydrating cream cleanser used in the morning to wash away the day's impurities, then use your toner.
Serum	At night, a retinol serum can help boost cell turnover and smooth fine lines, which is especially beneficial for menopausal skin. If retinol doesn't suit you, try a firming peptide serum or a nourishing ceramide-based formula instead. Choose what works best for your skin
Night Cream	Choose a rich, nourishing night cream that hydrates deeply while you sleep.
Eye Cream	Finish your evening routine with an eye cream to keep the under-eye area hydrated and smooth.
Neck Cream	Apply a neck cream to improve your skin's texture and firmness and for hydration overnight.

Using your regular cleanser around the eyes can actually contribute to puffiness and irritation, especially during menopause when the skin becomes more sensitive. Eye makeup removers are specially formulated to be gentle on this delicate area, helping to avoid unnecessary swelling or dryness that menopause can already intensify.

"Your skin is the largest organ in your body: Often overlooked, the skin isn't just a protective barrier but a dynamic organ that plays a vital role in temperature regulation, immunity and sensation."

Starting Small

If you're not used to using a lot of skincare products, don't feel like you need to do everything at once. Start small! Begin with a good cleanser and day cream with SPF and build from there as you feel more comfortable. Do what works for you. There's no need to have an elaborate routine unless it suits your lifestyle. Keep it simple and effective! Remembering to do it every day is the most important thing - it should feel like brushing your teeth, a habit that you don't even think about, you just do it.

Screens and Skin Ageing – What You Need to Know

Something that's come to light more recently is the impact our digital lives can have on our skin. We often don't realise how much time we spend in front of screens, but the blue light emitted from phones, tablets and computers can contribute to premature ageing. It penetrates deeper than UV rays, accelerating skin damage that can lead to fine lines, wrinkles, dryness, sensitivity and even pigmentation.

It's not just about the light itself. The constant posture we hold while looking at screens can add to skin concerns, especially around the neck and jawline. Add in the eye strain, which can make us squint and frown and it all shows up on our skin.

The good news? You can take steps to reduce the damage. Take regular breaks from screens, use blue light filters and choose skincare with antioxidants and SPF 30+ for added protection. It's a modern challenge, but with a few mindful tweaks, you can help keep your skin looking its best.

"Don't use your regular day or night cream around your eyes, as it can cause irritation or puffiness. The skin in this area is much thinner and more delicate, particularly during menopause, so it requires a lighter, specially formulated eye cream to provide proper care and hydration."

Targeting Menopause-Specific Skin Concerns

How we experience this transition through menopause is individual and how this affects our skin is also different for everyone. During menopause, your skin changes in ways you might not expect, often leading to new or intensified skin issues. These changes are largely due to fluctuating hormone levels, especially the drop in oestrogen and progesterone, which can impact the skin's hydration, elasticity and overall appearance. You can feel like your skin has lost its glow. Here, we'll explore some of the most common skin concerns you may face during menopause and how you can address them with home products and salon treatments.

Daily sunscreen is your skin's best defence against ageing.

---

1. Fine Lines and Wrinkles

As your skin produces less collagen and elastin, fine lines and wrinkles may become more noticeable, particularly around the eyes, mouth, neck and forehead area.

What helps?

Incorporate a retinol or retinoid (a form of Vitamin A) into your routine. Retinol is one of my favourite ingredients because it encourages skin cell turnover and stimulates collagen production, helping to reduce the appearance of wrinkles. There are different types of retinoids as discussed earlier in this chapter.

Salon Treatments:

Micro-needling, laser resurfacing, microdermabrasion or chemical peels can all help reduce fine lines and wrinkles by encouraging the skin to regenerate and produce more collagen.

2. Dryness

The skin becomes drier as you age but oestrogen also plays a key role in maintaining skin hydration. As it declines during menopause, your skin may feel drier than before.

What helps?

Hyaluronic acid is a powerful humectant that draws moisture into the skin, while ceramides help to lock that moisture in, keeping your skin hydrated. Use a good night cream and serum with these ingredients and don't forget to drink plenty of water to keep your skin hydrated from within. At home hydrating masks and peels can help keep the skin hydrated.

Salon Treatments

Deep hydrating facials, gentle chemical peels (like those using AHAs) and advanced treatments such as Hydra facials can give your skin a much-needed moisture boost and smoother texture. To support this at home, try adding a hydrating mask once or twice a week to keep your skin soft, plump and glowing.

3. Loss of Elasticity and Sagging

Reduced collagen production can lead to sagging skin, particularly around the jawline and neck.

What helps?

Using peptide-based serums can stimulate collagen production, helping to firm the skin. Collagen-boosting products such as retinol can also improve elasticity.

Salon Treatments:

Radiofrequency skin tightening, ultrasound therapy and collagen-inducing facials can help improve skin elasticity and reduce sagging.

4. Hyperpigmentation (Dark Spots)

Menopausal skin can be more prone to hyperpigmentation or dark spots due to sun exposure and hormonal changes.

What helps?

Vitamin C serums are excellent for brightening the skin and fading dark spots. Products with AHAs (alpha hydroxy acids) can also help to exfoliate the skin and reduce pigmentation. And always apply a sunscreen SPF 30+ every day of the year!

Salon Treatments:

Chemical peels or laser treatments are effective options for tackling hyperpigmentation at a deeper level. Micro needling and microdermabrasion are also helpful for pigmentation.

5. Itchy, Sensitive Skin

What Helps?

Opt for fragrance-free, gentle cleansers and moisturisers. Look for products containing soothing ingredients like aloe vera, chamomile, or colloidal oatmeal, which help calm irritated skin. Applying body lotion or oil immediately after showering can help lock in moisture and reduce itchiness.

I often recommend Garshana gloves to my clients. These silk exfoliating gloves, traditionally used in Ayurvedic practices, are a lovely way to gently dry brush the skin before showering. They help slough off dead skin cells, boost circulation and improve how well your skincare products absorb. This simple ritual can leave your skin feeling softer, more hydrated and can also ease the itchiness that often comes with drier menopausal skin.

Salon Treatments:

If your skin feels particularly dry and irritated, professional treatments can provide relief. Soothing body treatments, such as hydrating wraps, gentle exfoliation treatments, or nourishing oil massages, can deeply moisturise and calm sensitive skin. Lymphatic drainage massages can also help improve circulation, reducing water retention and improving skin texture.

For the face, hydrating facials with calming ingredients can soothe irritation and strengthen the skin barrier. If you experience dryness or flaking, ask your therapist about treatments like oxygen facials, LED light therapy, or hyaluronic acid-infused masks to replenish hydration and restore your skin's natural glow.

6. Skin Tags

These irritating pieces of skin can suddenly appear, often around the neck and underarm area, though they can develop anywhere. While harmless, they can be annoying or unsightly. The good news is that a dermatologist or qualified practitioner can easily remove skin tags using methods like freezing, diathermy or cauterising.

7. Oestrogen, Vitamin D and your Skin

Oestrogen plays a crucial role in skin health by stimulating the enzyme responsible for activating vitamin D in the skin. Vitamin D, in its active form, is essential for maintaining the skin's barrier function, promoting cell turnover and supporting overall skin health.

When oestrogen levels decline during menopause, this activation process can slow down, potentially leading to vitamin D deficiency. This may contribute to dryness, reduced elasticity and a compromised skin barrier.

What helps?

Get Outside: Spend some time in sunlight daily if you can, to boost natural vitamin D production, just avoid prolonged exposure without SPF.

Eat Well: Include vitamin D-rich foods such as salmon, eggs, mushrooms and fortified options in your diet.

Consider Supplements: Taking a vitamin D supplement may be beneficial, especially during winter or in areas with limited sunlight.

Menopausal skin concerns are common, but they aren't always spoken about as much as the more classic symptoms like hot flushes. If you are experiencing changes in your skin it doesn't have to leave you feeling helpless.

By choosing the right products and, if professional treatments are your thing, you can help your skin stay healthy, firm and glowing throughout menopause. Whether it's adding a retinol to your nightly routine or treating yourself to a hydrating facial (which is also very relaxing), small steps can make a big difference. It's all about prevention and preserving what you've got.

Professional Beauty Treatments for Menopausal Skin

Professional treatments aren't for everyone, but when combined with a good at-home skincare routine, they can make a real difference in addressing some of the skin concerns that come with menopause. As women, we often feel guilty about spending time or money on ourselves but this is exactly the time in life when we need to prioritise our own care, not put it on the back burner.

These treatments not only help to improve the condition and appearance of your skin, but they also offer a deeply relaxing, restorative experience which is a powerful tool for reducing stress. Menopause can bring dryness, sensitivity, loss of elasticity and more visible fine lines and wrinkles, but there are now so many targeted, evidence-based options to support your skin through these changes.

Here are a few professional treatments worth considering to support your skin's health and help you feel your best.

1. Hydrating Facials

Menopausal skin often experiences dryness due to a decrease in oestrogen, which affects the skin's ability to retain moisture. Hydrating facials are designed to deeply moisturise and nourish the skin, using ingredients like hyaluronic acid to help lock in hydration. One treatment I often recommend is the HydraFacial, a popular, non-invasive facial that combines cleansing, exfoliation, hydration and antioxidant infusion all in one.

What it does: These facials work to replenish lost moisture and revitalise tired, dull-looking skin.

Why it helps: When your skin is properly hydrated, it appears plumper, smoother and more radiant, helping to soften the appearance of fine lines and restore a healthy glow.

2. Collagen-Boosting Treatments

As we age, our skin's collagen production declines, leading to sagging and loss of firmness. Collagen-boosting treatments, like microneedling or radiofrequency, work to stimulate the skin's natural collagen production.

What it does: These treatments help firm the skin and reduce the appearance of fine lines and wrinkles by encouraging collagen regeneration.

Why it helps: Boosting collagen production helps restore some of the skin's natural elasticity, making it look firmer and more youthful.

3. Chemical Peels

Chemical peels can be a great option for addressing multiple menopausal skin concerns, including hyperpigmentation, dullness and uneven skin tone. Peels remove the outer layer of skin, revealing fresh, brighter skin underneath.

What it does: By using acids like glycolic or lactic acid, a chemical peel gently exfoliates the skin to promote cell turnover.

Why it helps: Regular chemical peels can help reduce dark spots, smooth fine lines, increase moisture levels and give the skin a more youthful glow.

4. Laser Treatments

Laser treatments, such as fractional lasers or intense pulsed light (IPL), are highly effective for targeting a range of issues from fine lines to sun damage and hyperpigmentation.

What it does: Lasers penetrate the skin to promote collagen production and target pigmentation at the surface level.

Why it helps: Laser treatments can help reduce the appearance of age spots, fine lines and promote a more even skin tone.

5. Radiofrequency Skin Tightening

Radiofrequency (RF) is a non-invasive treatment that uses heat to stimulate collagen and elastin production, tightening the skin and reducing the appearance of fine lines.

What it does: RF helps to lift and tighten sagging skin, particularly around the jawline and neck area, which can be areas of concern during menopause.

Why it helps: By tightening the skin without the need for surgery, this treatment can offer a natural-looking lift and more defined contours.

6. Oxygen Therapy Facials

Oxygen therapy is another popular treatment that infuses the skin with oxygen and active ingredients to boost hydration and reduce signs of ageing.

What it does: The oxygen delivery system hydrates the skin, plumps it up and promotes cell turnover.

Why it helps: Oxygen facials can immediately give the skin a boost, leaving it brighter and more youthful looking.

7. LED Light Therapy

LED light therapy uses different wavelengths of light to target specific skin issues, such as fine lines, inflammation and dullness.

What it does: The light penetrates the skin to help reduce inflammation, stimulate collagen production and improve overall skin tone.

Why it helps: It's a non-invasive, pain-free treatment that's great for all skin types and is particularly helpful for calming sensitive or irritated menopausal skin.

These treatments, when paired with a good at-home skincare routine, can dramatically improve the appearance and feel of your menopausal skin. Professional therapies can provide that extra boost your skin needs during this phase of life, helping you feel confident and radiant.

Remember, it's not just about addressing the visible signs of ageing but about taking care of your skin's health and well-being. Before undergoing any professional treatment, consult with a qualified beauty therapist to determine the best options for your specific concerns.

Nourish Your Skin – The Best Foods for a Healthy, Glowing Complexion

When it comes to skin, I simply can't leave out nutrition, it's far too important. Yes, using high-quality products and having the right treatments matter, but what you eat is just as vital. Your skin needs the right nutrients to truly thrive. And during menopause, when hormonal shifts are already affecting your skin's appearance and behaviour, nourishing yourself from the inside becomes even more important.

I've worked with so many women who struggled with dullness, breakouts, acne, dryness or flare-ups during menopause and in many cases, nutrition was the missing piece. Once we cleaned up their diets and added in a few key nutrients, their skin started to change. That glow returned, the sensitivity settled, and they felt better all over.

I know this from personal experience too. I battled acne as a teenager, and even back then, I realised food was part of the puzzle. I changed my diet and saw a big difference not an easy decision when you're young and surrounded by junk food! But it taught me early on that what we put in our bodies shows up on our skin.

In this section, I'll share the key nutrients and foods that can help support radiant, healthy skin through menopause and beyond. It's about giving your skin the building blocks it needs from the inside out.

Client Story: The Missing Piece

Years ago, when I was working as a beauty therapist, a client came to me struggling with perimenopausal acne. We started a course of treatments and adjusted her skincare routine at home. Over time, we saw noticeable improvements, but not quite the results I had hoped for.

After about six weeks of not seeing her, she returned and I was amazed, her skin looked incredible. The acne was gone and she had a beautiful glow. Naturally, I asked her what she had done. Her answer was simple: "I went to see a nutritional therapist and changed my diet."

It was a powerful reminder that what we put into our bodies is just as important as what we put on our skin. Nutrition is often the missing piece when it comes to achieving truly healthy, radiant skin.

What Does Your Skin Need?

Here is a table for the key vitamins and minerals that can be helpful for your skin as it ages, during menopause and beyond.

Ingredient	What it does	Where to find it
Vitamin C	Boosts collagen production, protects against sun damage and helps to brighten the skin.	Citrus fruits (oranges, lemons), strawberries, bell peppers, broccoli, and spinach.
Vitamin E	Acts as a powerful antioxidant, protecting skin cells from free radical damage and helping to maintain skin moisture.	Nuts and seeds (almonds, sunflower seeds), spinach and avocados,
Vitamin A	Essential for cell turnover, helping to reduce wrinkles and maintain healthy skin tone. It's also crucial in the form of retinol for anti-ageing.	Sweet potatoes, carrots, spinach and good old liver which fewer people eat these days.
Vitamin D	Helps with skin cell growth, repair and metabolism. It's also	Fatty fish (salmon, mackerel), fortified dairy products and

	anti-inflammatory.	sunlight exposure.
Zinc	Reduces inflammation and speeds up skin healing. It's essential for healthy oil production in the skin.	Pumpkin seeds, chickpeas, lentils and whole grains.
Omega-3 Fatty Acids	Helps to maintain skin's lipid barrier, reducing dryness and keeping skin hydrated.	Fatty fish (salmon, mackerel, herring), flaxseeds, walnuts and chia seeds.
Biotin (Vitamin B7)	Supports the health of skin, hair and nails by promoting cell production and growth.	Eggs, almonds, sweet potatoes and whole grains.
Selenium	Acts as a powerful antioxidant, helping to protect skin from environmental damage and inflammation.	Brazil nuts, fish, eggs and brown rice.

Targeted Nutrition for Common Skin Concerns During Menopause

Issue	Nutrient	Sources
1. Dry Skin During menopause, your skin's ability to retain moisture diminishes.	Vitamin E helps maintain the skin's moisture barrier and prevents dryness.	Almonds, sunflower seeds, spinach.
	Omega-3 Fatty Acids are essential for keeping skin hydrated by maintaining the lipid barrier.	Salmon, chia seeds, flaxseeds.
	Vitamin D supports skin cell growth and repair, which can help with moisture retention.	Fatty fish, fortified dairy products, and sunlight.
2. Wrinkles and Fine Lines As collagen levels drop during menopause, wrinkles and fine lines become more prominent.	Vitamin C boosts collagen production, helping to reduce the appearance of wrinkles.	Oranges, strawberries, broccoli.
	Vitamin A (Retinol) encourages cell turnover and helps reduce fine lines.	Carrots, sweet potatoes, spinach.

	Collagen supports skin elasticity and firmness.	Bone broth, collagen supplements, fish skin.
3. Sagging Skin Sagging is common as collagen production declines with age.	Collagen replenishes lost collagen to improve firmness.	Collagen supplements, bone broth, fish skin.
	Vitamin C supports the formation of new collagen.	Bell peppers, citrus fruits, kiwis.
4. Pigmentation and Age Spots Hormonal changes can lead to pigmentation issues.	Vitamin C brightens skin and fades pigmentation by reducing melanin production.	Citrus fruits, tomatoes, strawberries.
	Vitamin E helps reduce hyperpigmentation and prevents UV damage.	Nuts, seeds, avocados.
5. Skin Sensitivity and Redness Menopause can make skin more sensitive.	Zinc has anti-inflammatory properties that calm sensitive, irritated skin.	Pumpkin seeds, chickpeas, cashews.
	Niacinamide (Vitamin B3) reduces inflammation and strengthens the skin's barrier.	Poultry, peanuts, brown rice.

6. Loss of Elasticity As skin loses elasticity, it becomes less firm.	Vitamin C stimulates collagen production, helping restore skin elasticity.	Oranges, berries, peppers.
	Vitamin A (Retinoids) helps with skin cell renewal and improves firmness.	Leafy greens, carrots, sweet potatoes.
7. Puffy Eyes Puffiness around the eyes is common as we age.	Vitamin K reduces puffiness and dark circles by improving circulation around the eyes.	Kale, spinach, broccoli.
	Iron prevents tired, puffy eyes by promoting proper blood circulation.	Lentils, spinach, tofu.
8. Itchy or Irritated Skin Itchy skin is often a frustrating symptom of menopause.	Omega-3 Fatty Acids reduce inflammation and soothe irritated skin.	Fish oils, flaxseeds, walnuts.
	Zinc helps soothe irritation and reduce itching.	Pumpkin seeds, whole grains.
9. Acne Hormonal shifts can also trigger acne during menopause.	Zinc reduces acne by regulating oil production and preventing bacterial infections.	Pumpkin seeds, oysters, lentils.

	Vitamin A (Retinoids) helps reduce acne formation by speeding up skin cell turnover.	Carrots, sweet potatoes, leafy greens.
	Vitamin E works as an antioxidant that helps heal skin and reduce scarring from acne.	Nuts, seeds, spinach.
	Omega-3 Fatty Acids reduce inflammation, which can decrease the severity of acne.	Fatty fish, chia seeds, flaxseeds.
	Selenium helps protect skin cells from damage and may improve acne by reducing inflammation.	Brazil nuts, eggs, sunflower seeds.
	Vitamin D helps modulate the immune response and reduce acne flare-ups.	Fortified dairy, sunlight, fatty fish.

Client story:

Jane's Journey to Healthier Skin at 49

Jane, 49, came to me with dry, irritated skin that had become much more sensitive since entering perimenopause. She was also dealing with puffiness and dark circles around her eyes, something she hadn't experienced before. Like many women, she felt frustrated and upset by these sudden skin changes.

We focused on improving her gut health by introducing anti-inflammatory foods such as leafy greens, berries and fatty fish into her diet. Additionally, Jane began drinking more water and included a collagen supplement powder in her daily routine. Alongside these nutritional changes, she adopted a consistent skincare routine at home, using gentle, hydrating products designed for sensitive skin.

Within a few weeks, Jane noticed that her skin felt less irritated, the puffiness around her eyes had reduced and her overall complexion seemed healthier. These simple, gradual changes helped her feel more comfortable in her skin and more in control of the change's menopause had brought.

Collagen and Menopausal Skin:
What You Need to Know

One question I get asked daily is what collagen supplements should I take and does it really work? Let's have a look at this and what the latest research is saying.

Collagen is a popular topic of conversation when it comes to menopausal skin, and I'm frequently asked about collagen supplements by my clients. As oestrogen levels decline during menopause, our natural collagen production slows down, leading to visible changes like wrinkles, sagging and dryness. So, let's take a closer look at what you need to know about collagen and how supplements may support your skin health during this stage of life.

Types of Collagen

Collagen is a protein that acts like the scaffolding for your skin, providing structure and elasticity. There are different types of collagen, but here are the three most relevant for skin health:

Type I: This is the most abundant collagen in the skin and is responsible for maintaining the structure and firmness of your skin.

Type II: Found in cartilage, this type is more related to joint health but may sometimes appear in supplements aimed at overall health.

Type III: Often found alongside Type I, it helps with skin elasticity and firmness.

Collagen Supplements

Many people consider taking collagen supplements to help replenish the body's natural supply. These supplements are typically made from animal sources, such as bovine (cow) or marine (fish), with marine collagen often being touted as better for skin due to its smaller molecules, making it easier for the body to absorb. When choosing a supplement, here are a few things to look out for:

Hydrolysed Collagen: This means the collagen has been broken down into smaller peptides, which makes it easier for your body to absorb and use.

Types of Collagen: Look for supplements that contain Type I and Type III collagen for skin benefits. These are the most relevant to skin health and elasticity.

Additives: Be mindful of additives, flavourings, or unnecessary fillers in the supplements. A clean, simple formulation is often best.

Do Collagen Supplements Work?

While research is ongoing, some studies suggest that taking collagen supplements can improve skin hydration, elasticity and reduce the appearance of wrinkles. Results vary and supplements tend to work best when taken consistently over a longer period.

What Else to Consider

Quality over Quantity: Not all collagen supplements are created equal, so look for high-quality sources. Marine collagen is often seen as more sustainable and better absorbed by the body.

Diet First: Remember, while supplements can help, a diet rich in collagen-boosting foods like bone broth, fish and vitamin C-rich fruits will also support your body's natural collagen production.

To summarise, while collagen supplements can be beneficial, they're not a magic solution on their own. Always ensure you're choosing a high-quality product that fits with your individual needs and combine it with a nutrient-rich diet to support your overall skin health. If you're unsure, consult with a healthcare provider to ensure it's the right choice for you.

Exploring Cosmetic Enhancements

Finally, I wanted to mention cosmetic enhancements, as they have in today's society become a common part of skincare for many women, particularly as we age and enter menopause. It's important to approach this topic without judgement, recognising that beauty and confidence are deeply personal. Each woman's choices are her own and feeling empowered in those decisions is what truly matters.

Injectable Enhancements

Botox: Reduces fine lines and wrinkles by relaxing targeted muscles, commonly used on areas like the forehead and around the eyes.

Dermal Fillers: Restores volume and contours to areas such as the cheeks and lips.

Skin Boosters (e.g., Profhilo, Restylane Skinboosters): Hydrates and improves skin elasticity, leaving a radiant finish.

Collagen Biostimulators (e.g., Sculptra): Stimulates natural collagen production to improve skin texture and gradually restore volume. Using poly-L-lactic acid (PLLA), a compound that triggers your body's own collagen production.

Polynucleotide Injections: A newer treatment that regenerates and repairs skin at a cellular level, enhancing tone and elasticity. Mesotherapy: Micro-injections of vitamins, enzymes and nutrients to rejuvenate and nourish the skin.

A Word of Caution

Cosmetic enhancements can provide excellent results when done safely by a professional but always consult a qualified and experienced doctor. Do thorough research, ask for recommendations and ensure the practitioner is certified in aesthetic treatments. Your safety and well-being should always come first.

Nurturing Your Nails and Hair Through Menopause

During menopause, hormonal changes can lead to noticeable shifts in hair and nail health. The decline in oestrogen not only reduces skin hydration but also affects the strength and resilience of hair and nails. Oestrogen plays a crucial role in maintaining collagen, a protein vital for the health of these areas. As levels drop, hair can become thinner, drier and more brittle, while nails may weaken and grow more slowly. Blood circulation may also decrease, affecting nutrient delivery to hair follicles and nail beds, which can contribute to this brittleness.

Though often overlooked, looking after your hair and nails during menopause can do wonders for confidence. Here are some simple, effective steps to help you keep them feeling strong, hydrated and healthy.

Strengthen Your Nails

Nails can become more fragile with hormonal shifts during menopause, particularly due to the decline in oestrogen levels that affects keratin production. These tips will help keep them strong and healthy.

Stay Hydrated: Regularly moisturise your hands and nails with a rich cream or cuticle oil to prevent splitting and peeling. For deeper hydration, use a hand mask at night by applying a nourishing cream and wearing thin cotton gloves to lock in moisture while you sleep.

Use SPF on Your Hands: Hands often show early signs of ageing due to daily sun exposure, yet they're easily overlooked. I always apply a little of my day cream with SPF to the backs of my hands after applying it to my face. It's a simple habit that can help prevent pigmentation and age spots.

Nourishing Nail Oil for Stronger Nails

Using a nail oil regularly can help hydrate and strengthen brittle nails, preventing peeling and breakage. Look for a blend that includes:

Jojoba oil – Absorbs well and deeply nourishes the nail and cuticles

Vitamin E oil – Promotes nail strength and resilience

Lavender essential oil – Hydrates and soothes dry, brittle nails

Myrrh essential oil – Helps prevent splitting and supports nail growth

Massage a few drops into your nails and cuticles daily for best results.

Exfoliate Regularly: Gently exfoliate your hands once a week to remove dead skin cells. This improves absorption for moisturisers and keeps the skin soft.

Give Nails a Break from Chemicals: Periodically go polish-free to let your nails breathe. When using polish, opt for non-toxic formulas that avoid harsh chemicals known to weaken nails.

Boost with Biotin: Biotin strengthens brittle nails. Consider a biotin supplement or add biotin-rich foods like eggs, almonds and sweet potatoes to your diet for natural support.

High-Tech, Breathable Nail Polishes

Traditional nail polishes can trap moisture and weaken nails, but new breathable polishes allow air and moisture to pass through, preventing dehydration and peeling while still providing colour and protection.

Limit Acetone-Based Nail Polish Removers

Harsh removers strip nails of moisture. Opt for acetone-free formulas or give your nails regular polish-free breaks to restore strength.

Aromatherapy for Nail Health: Lavender essential oil can help nourish and protect nails, especially during menopause when hormonal changes can lead to dryness and brittleness. Add a few drops to your hand cream for an extra boost of moisture and soothing care.

Supporting Hair Health

This is an area I certainly noticed when I hit perimenopause. It felt like my hair thinned out overnight! The truth is, as oestrogen levels decline, the hair's growth cycle can be disrupted, leading to increased shedding, thinning, or slower regrowth. Many women also notice their hair becomes drier or more brittle, especially around the hairline or crown.

What many don't realise is that testosterone also influences hair growth. Women naturally produce small amounts of testosterone, which helps stimulate hair follicles and maintain hair density. But during menopause, levels of both oestrogen and testosterone can decline and when testosterone drops too low, it may contribute to thinner, slower-growing hair. On the flip side, if testosterone becomes dominant relative to oestrogen, some women may notice hair thinning at the crown and unwanted facial hair.

Hormonal shifts can also affect the scalp's oil production, making hair feel less glossy, while changes in nutrient absorption can affect its strength and texture.

The good news is there's a lot you can do from eating a nutrient-rich diet and using scalp-supportive products to managing stress and considering targeted supplementation, to help support your hair.

Nourish with Omega-3s: Essential fatty acids found in foods like salmon, chia seeds, and walnuts help maintain scalp health and support hair growth. Consider an omega-3 supplement if you're not getting enough from your diet.

Weekly Hair Mask: Treat your hair to a hydrating mask once a week. Look for masks with ingredients like keratin, coconut oil or shea butter to add moisture, strength and shine.

Nourish Your Scalp and Hair with Oils: A scalp massage with nourishing oils can boost circulation, stimulate hair follicles and promote healthy growth. Try massaging a few drops of diluted rosemary or lavender oil into your scalp; rosemary stimulates hair growth and lavender provides hydration and a calming effect.

For added softness and shine, use a hair oil like argan oil on the ends of your hair after styling or as an overnight treatment. Always dilute essential oils with a carrier oil, such as jojoba or sweet almond oil, or choose a pre-mixed blend for easy application.

Consider Collagen: Collagen supports both skin and hair health by providing essential amino acids. A daily scoop of collagen powder can help strengthen hair, enhancing resilience and thickness.

Keep Expectations Realistic

Finally, remember that changes to nails and hair won't happen overnight. Patience is key, small, daily actions add up over time. It's about embracing your natural beauty and making the most of what you have. With a little extra care, you can keep both your nails and hair looking vibrant and strong as you navigate this stage of life.

Supplements to Consider for Hair and Nails

- **Collagen Peptides (Type I & III)** – Supports skin elasticity, hydration and firmness. Also strengthens nails and hair. Best absorbed when taken with vitamin C.

- **Sea Buckthorn Oil (Omega-7)** – Deeply hydrates skin and mucous membranes (vaginal, oral, nasal). Supports skin regeneration, elasticity and soothes dryness linked to oestrogen decline.

- **Omega-3 Fatty Acids (EPA & DHA)** – Reduces skin inflammation, supports barrier function, and improves hydration. Also beneficial for hormonal balance and calming reactive skin.

- **Vitamin C** – Essential for collagen synthesis, skin repair and brightening. Helps reduce pigmentation and oxidative stress that accelerates ageing.

- **Zinc** – Supports wound healing, regulates oil production, calms acne and strengthens the skin barrier. Also promotes healthy nail growth and reduces irritation.

- **Evening Primrose Oil (GLA)** – Helps soothe dry, itchy, or sensitive skin by improving moisture retention

- **Biotin (Vitamin B7)** – Supports keratin production in skin, hair and nails. May help improve brittle nails and support thicker hair growth.

- **Vitamin D3** – Aids skin cell turnover and barrier repair. Low levels are linked to dryness, inflammation and reduced healing capacity, especially post-menopause.

- **Iron (if deficient)** – Iron deficiency is strongly linked to hair thinning and shedding. Always test before supplementing.

- **Saw Palmetto** – Can be helpful for women with androgenic hair loss (thinning at the crown), as it blocks the conversion of testosterone to DHT, which can damage hair follicles. Often used in combination with zinc and biotin.

Three Quick Wins

1. Apply your day cream with SPF to the backs of your hands as well as your face every morning to help prevent age spots and sun damage.

2. Exfoliate your body three to four times a week with Garshana gloves to ease dry, itchy skin and improve glow and product absorption.

3. Use a proper eye makeup remover not your facial cleanser to avoid puffiness and irritation around the delicate eye area, especially during menopause when skin becomes more sensitive.

---

11 CREATING CONSISTENCY –
THE KEY TO LONG-TERM WELLNESS

"The smallest habits, done regularly,
are what truly create long-term change."

Alison Bladh

Five Things You'll Learn in this Chapter:

- Why **small, consistent habits** are more effective than all-or-nothing efforts

- How to **anchor new habits** into your existing routine with ease

- Ways to **use habit stacking** to make change feel effortless

- How to **overcome common barriers** like low energy, lack of time, or overwhelm

- **The power of tracking** and celebrating progress even on the tough days

---

As we age and move through different life phases, especially during menopause! Building and maintaining routines can feel overwhelming. When you're already dealing with fatigue, fluctuating hormones, work, family and the constant demands of daily life, self-care can easily feel like just another task on an already packed to-do list.

But what if we looked at wellness through a different lens? Instead of trying to change everything at once, what if we focused on small, meaningful habits that energise us, boost our confidence and bring clarity rather than drain what little energy we have left?

Now that we've explored so many essential aspects of wellness throughout the book, this chapter is about weaving them together in a way that feels realistic, manageable and sustainable so the changes you've started don't just stick, they support you for life.

And it all starts with a decision.

Not a huge, overwhelming one. Not a "I'll start Monday" kind of decision. Just a simple choice to show up for yourself today. To take one small step in the direction you want to go.

Because here's the truth: change doesn't happen all at once. It's the small things, done consistently, that create real, lasting results.

Decisions are powerful. Every choice we make, no matter how small, shapes the direction of our lives. We often think we need the perfect plan, the perfect moment, or the perfect motivation to start but that's not true. The power lies in deciding.

Right now, you have the power to decide to take care of yourself. You don't have to wait until you feel ready. You don't need permission. The smallest decision choosing to drink more water today, to take a five-minute walk, to go to bed a little earlier can be the start of something bigger.

Ask yourself: "What's one small decision you can make today that will help you feel better tomorrow?"

This chapter is about discovering how small steps, done gradually, with compassion, can become the foundation of a wellness approach that lasts a lifetime. Staying consistent is less about being perfect and more about showing up for yourself, even if it's just for five minutes.

You don't need to get it right every day, you just need to keep going.

As you move through this chapter, think about what changes feel doable for you. The habits that fit your life, your energy, your priorities. It's not about following a rigid plan; it's about creating a lifestyle that works for you.

Because in the end, the most powerful changes aren't the biggest, they're the ones you decide to stick with.

Building Habits that Stick

Staying consistent with your health and wellness routines can feel like an uphill climb especially when you're already juggling responsibilities and navigating hormonal changes. I get it. A new wellness plan often starts out feeling exciting, but after a week or two, the motivation fades and life quickly takes over. What I've learned is that lasting change doesn't come from all-or-nothing efforts. It comes from small, steady actions that quietly build momentum and lead to something powerful.

The beauty of small, consistent actions is that they don't drain us, they give us a boost, even when we're feeling low on energy. Think of wellness habits like planting seeds. At first, you might not see much change. But with each small effort, you're nurturing something that grows stronger and more beautiful over time. Building habits that last is about making a commitment to yourself in a way that feels manageable, kind and forgiving and most importantly, joyful. Having worked with clients for many years, I can honestly say the hardest part for most people is making the change, putting new things into practice on a daily basis. We are creatures of habit! And even when we have the best intentions in the world and are really motivated it can be hard to make that habit stick; and when our motivation wanes (which it will do in the long term) we find ourselves going back to the old 'not so healthy' habits we had before.

So, let's keep it simple. Here are three ways to start building habits that can truly stick:

Anchor Habits: Start with something so simple it feels almost too easy. This could be drinking a glass of water as soon as you wake up or taking a few deep breaths before starting your day. Think of these as anchor points, small actions you can rely on, no matter how busy things get. Anchoring habits act as a standalone foundation, easy to do and set the tone for the day. Once you've got one or two of these anchors in place, you can gradually build on them with additional wellness actions.

Anchor Habit Examples:

Building Consistency with Simple, Standalone Actions

Before you get out of bed, take a quiet moment to pause and breathe deeply. Just a few slow breaths can calm your nervous system, clear your mind and help you start the day feeling centred and grounded.

Habit	Action
Daily Five-Minute Journal Reflection	Keep a notebook by your bedside and jot down one sentence each evening about your day. It could be something you accomplished, a gratitude statement, or simply a thought about tomorrow. This daily pause encourages a sense of accomplishment and mindfulness. Example: "I handled a stressful moment calmly today and I'm proud of that."
One Nutrient-Dense Snack Daily	Select a time in your day to enjoy a nutrient-packed snack, like a small handful of nuts with a piece of fruit. By anchoring this to a time (like mid-morning), you can more easily work in healthy nutrients that support energy and mood, without requiring a big dietary overhaul.
Gentle Stretch Before Bed	Spend a few minutes each night doing gentle stretching, focusing on areas that may feel tense. This can help relax your muscles and prepare your body for rest.
Afternoon Energy Reset	Around mid-afternoon, take a brief pause to step outside, even if it's just on the balcony or garden. A

	breath of fresh air and a change of scenery helps to rejuvenate energy and shift perspective.
Breathing Pause before Each Meal	Before starting a meal, take three deep breaths. This grounding practice aids digestion and can reduce stress.
Set a daily "Wellness alarm"	Set an alarm at the same time each day as a reminder to check in with yourself. When the alarm goes off, take a moment to ask, "How am I feeling at the moment?" and do a quick scan of your body and mind.
Pre-Bed Reflection Ritual	Each night before bed, take a quiet moment to think of one thing you're looking forward to tomorrow. This gentle focus on something positive helps end your day with hope. If anything is on your mind or causing worry, write it down to ease mental clutter and support more restful sleep.
Dedicated hydration habit	Choose a time in the day, like in the morning first thing or right after lunch, to drink a full glass of water. Anchoring hydration to a specific time helps maintain a healthy water intake with minimal effort.

A client told me how adding five minutes of deep breathing daily improved her sleep and now she wakes up with less puffiness and brighter skin!

Habit Stacking

This is one of my favourites and I have seen it work well with clients. My dumbbells by the kettle that I mentioned in chapter 9 is a good example for this. One of the easiest ways to add new habits is to stack them onto something you're already doing. For example, if you're already making tea or coffee in the morning, use that time to do a few stretches, a deep breathing exercise, or set your intentions for the day. Habit stacking makes new routines feel natural because they're linked to things you're already doing.

"You don't need a complete overhaul. You need a gentle, steady rhythm that supports your life not complicates it."

Alison Bladh

Simple Habit Stacking Ideas for Busy Women

Habit Stack	Action
Morning Hydration with Affirmations	While drinking your first glass of water of the day, take a moment to think of one positive intention for the day. This can be as simple as "I'm taking care of myself" or "Today, I'm going to have a nice healthy lunch."
Stretch While Brushing Your Teeth	Use the two minutes of brushing to do gentle stretches like calf raises. It's a quick way to get a bit of movement into your day.
Deep Breaths While Waiting for the Kettle	When waiting for your kettle to boil or brewing your coffee, try three deep, intentional breaths to centre yourself. This simple practice can reduce stress and bring a moment of calm into your morning.
Kitchen Counter Push-Ups	Turn your kitchen counter into a mini gym! Place your hands on the edge of the counter or against the wall, step your feet back and do a few push-ups. It's a simple way to strengthen your

	arms and chest while waiting for food to cook.
Side Leg Lifts While Washing Up	Turn dishwashing into a balance challenge! Stand on one leg and slowly lift the other leg out to the side. Lower it back down with control, then switch sides. This simple move strengthens your hips, improves balance and adds a bit of fun to your kitchen routine.
Peel your skin while in the shower	While showering, use a body brush or exfoliating mitts in light, circular motions to boost circulation, remove dead skin cells and encourage smoother, more radiant skin. This simple practice also supports lymphatic flow and may help improve the appearance of cellulite.
Easy veggie boost	When having lunch or dinner, add a handful of fresh veggies like spinach or tomatoes. This simple habit instantly boosts your meal with fibre and nutrients, supporting steady energy and overall wellness.

Walk and talk	If you have calls you need to make, try taking them on a walk. Walking while chatting is a great way to get fresh air and steps without adding extra time to your schedule.
Shoulder rolls while waiting for the microwave	Use the minute or two waiting for food to heat up to gently roll your shoulders and release tension, especially if you've been working at a desk.
Gratitude practice at bedtime	When climbing into bed, think of one thing you're grateful for from the day. This helps end the day on a positive note and reinforces self-care as a natural part of your routine.
Hand cream and mindfulness	After washing your hands, take a moment to massage the hand cream slowly. Use this as a brief mindfulness exercise, paying attention to each finger as you apply, while hydrating and caring for your skin.
Core engagement while sitting	When you're sitting at your desk, in the car, or waiting somewhere, take a few moments to engage

	your core muscles. Sit up straight, gently pull in your stomach and hold for a few breaths.

These small, manageable habits fit into everyday moments, making them easy to keep up and helping you weave wellness into your day without added stress.

Track Your Progress

Tracking isn't for everyone. Some find it motivating, while others prefer a more flexible approach. But for many of my clients, it's a simple yet effective way to stay on track. Whether it's ticking off a calendar, using an app or jotting a quick note in a journal, having a visual record of your efforts can be incredibly encouraging. It helps you see the progress you're making, even if it's just one small step at a time. And on the days that feel hard, you'll have proof that you still did something good for yourself and that's worth celebrating.

"Habits are the compound interest of self-improvement. The same way that money multiplies through compound interest, the effects of your habits multiply as you repeat them."

James Clear (taken from Atomic Habits)

Building Habits That Last

Consistency is a muscle you build over time and it's okay if it takes a while to get there. Just know that these small, manageable steps are your foundation. With each one, you're building a stronger, more resilient version of yourself, ready to embrace your wellness for the long term. Two of my favourite books on habits and habit change are Atomic Habits by James Clear and Tiny Habits by JG Fogg - both well worth a read if you want to dig deeper into the world of habits.

You might be wondering, "How long does it actually take to build a new habit?" The truth is, it varies. Some habits take longer to stick than others, and it really depends on the person and the complexity of the habit. Research by Dr Phillippa Lally and her team at University College London, published in the European Journal of Social Psychology, found that it takes an average of 66 days for a new behaviour to become automatic but the range was anywhere from 18 to 254 days.

Experts like James Clear, author of Atomic Habits, remind us that it's not really about the number of days it's about repetition and consistency. The more often you do something, and the easier you make it, the more likely it is to become part of your routine.

So, while we often hear about the 21-day or 30-day habit myths, real change usually takes a bit longer and that's okay. What matters most is that you keep going and make those habits manageable and realistic for you.

> Research shows it's often the small, repeated actions that shape our lives the most. For example, making just a 1% improvement every day adds up to nearly 38% growth over a year. Small steps create remarkable progress when they're done consistently.

Overcoming Common Barriers to Consistency

When it comes to building a wellness routine, staying consistent is often the hardest part. Between a packed schedule, fluctuating moods and energy levels and the usual disruptions of daily life, it's easy to feel like wellness habits take a back seat. But by identifying the common barriers that get in the way, you can create practical solutions that make it easier to stay on track, even during busy times.

Barrier 1: Feeling Short on Time

One of the biggest challenges I see among clients is the belief that wellness takes too much time. But the truth is, small actions or baby steps make a big difference. A 'movement snack' like stretching while the kettle boils or a few squats while you brush your teeth are simple ways to stay active without setting aside a dedicated hour. And it doesn't stop at movement! Wellness snippets can be beauty and nutrition-based, too like adding a handful of greens to lunch or an extra glass of water before each meal is a small action that can support your energy levels and skin hydration. You could also try some face yoga while waiting for the water to run warm, for example, gently puff out your cheeks with air and hold for a few seconds, then release. This helps tone facial muscles and improves circulation.

Practical Tip: Try setting a five minute 'wellness window' into your morning and evening routine. Use this time to stretch, take deep breaths, apply a moisturising serum, or go for a quick walk. These short bursts are powerful and can fit into almost any schedule, supporting both inner and outer wellness.

Barrier 2: Low energy or motivation

During menopause and the years surrounding it, energy levels can be unpredictable, to say the least. On days when energy is low, think about finding activities that work with your energy, not against it. Gentle stretches, a calming walk, or even deep breathing exercises can re-energise you without demanding too much effort. And if you're needing a quick nutrient boost, a small snack rich in healthy fats or a few nuts can help lift your energy without a blood sugar spike, keeping your wellness going even on tougher days.

Practical Tip: Write a 'low-energy day' list with simple wellness ideas like stretching, a five-minute walk, breathing in some aromatherapy oils, applying a facemask, breathing exercises, or sipping a green tea that you can pull from on days when motivation feels low. This keeps wellness accessible, even when you're not feeling your best.

Barrier 3: Forgetting new habits

New habits can slip your mind, especially when routines aren't fully established. Habit stacking by adding a wellness activity to something you're already doing can help keep you consistent. For example, if you're brushing your teeth or making tea, that's your cue to do a quick stretch, spray your skin with a hydrating mist, or set a daily intention. By pairing wellness habits with daily actions, these habits become automatic over time and fit effortlessly into your routine.

Practical Tip: Set up visual reminders around your home, like a water bottle by your favourite chair or a moisturiser beside your bedside table. These small cues help make wellness a regular, easy-to-remember part of your day.

Barrier 4: Information overload

I really get it. There is so much information and misinformation out there it's enough to stress anyone out at the best of times! With so much conflicting advice on health and wellness during menopause, it's easy to feel overwhelmed and unsure where to start. This overload can lead to indecision, preventing you from taking any action at all. For women dealing with life changes and menopause, sifting through endless tips can be frustrating and really demotivating.

Practical Tip: Start with one reliable source, such as a book (like this one!) or a trusted professional and implement just one small change at a time. Keeping it simple can help cut through the noise, making the process manageable and enjoyable.

Barrier 5: The 'I'll Start on Monday' Trap

It's so easy to fall into the pattern of seeing Monday as a fresh start, a little 'New Year' each week where we promise ourselves that this time, we'll stick to all the wellness goals. But this mindset often turns today into a free pass to overindulge, while we push any real action to 'next Monday' when we'll suddenly be ready for squats, long walks and kale salads. Sound familiar?

Practical Tip: Try to ditch the Monday mindset. Take one small action today, just do it! even if it's just five minutes of stretching or adding extra veggies to your dinner. Wellness habits can start any day, at any time you don't need a fresh calendar week to make progress.

Consistency isn't about doing the same thing perfectly every day. It's about finding what works, making small adjustments and giving yourself grace along the way. By removing common barriers, you're building a foundation of wellness that can grow with you, regardless of menopause and life's ups and downs. In the next part, we'll look at strategies for tracking your progress and celebrating small wins because each step you take is one step closer to long-term wellness.

"You don't need to wait for Monday to change your life, just start with one small step today."

Alison Bladh

Creating a wellness routine for life

Now, I'm going to bring everything together and show you a wellness guide that integrates all the elements we've explored so far, demonstrating how achievable wellness is with a step-by-step approach. By viewing wellness as a practice rather than a checklist, you can create a lifestyle that doesn't require perfection but values consistency, self-compassion and flexibility. Your wellness plan is meant to be as unique as you are, tailored to support your body, mind and appearance through menopause and beyond. Small, consistent steps can lead to meaningful, lasting changes, so feel free to personalise this guide and make it truly yours.

"We should always be making space for wellness;
it should be something that is so automatic
that we don't even have to think about it."

Serena Williams

Client Story:
Small Steps Lead to a Big Change

Karen, 48 was a client who came to me struggling to stick to her health and wellness routines. "I start strong, but life always gets in the way," she says.

We focused on simple, consistent habits. She began with a glass of water each morning and stretching for two minutes while waiting for dinner to cook. Over time, she added a short evening walk and a gratitude journal before bed.

"These small changes didn't feel overwhelming," Karen shared later. "They fit into my life and actually stuck. I finally feel like I'm taking care of myself."

Karen's journey shows that lasting wellness isn't about perfection it's about finding small, doable steps that build consistency and momentum.

Your Wellness Plan in Practice:
Feel Great Every Day, Putting It All Together

This is a flexible example for structuring your weekly wellness plan. Adapt each day to suit your energy, preferences and wellness goals.

You'll find your Wellness Promise Planner and a QR code to download your own copy on page 376.

Day: Monday	
Movement	Gentle morning stretches
Nutrition	Add extra vegetables to lunch or dinner
Beauty/ Skincare	Hydrate skin with a soothing face mist during the day. Have it on your desk at work.
Mindset/ Stress Reduction	Take five minutes for deep breathing
Extra	Set an intention for the week
Day: Tuesday	
Movement	Brisk 20-min walk
Nutrition	Drink a glass of water before each meal
Beauty/ Skincare	Use a gentle exfoliator in the shower. Dry body brushing is great and so easy to do.
Mindset/ Stress Reduction	Write down one thing you're grateful for
Sleep Support	Avoid screens an hour before bed or wear blue light blocking glasses

Day: Wednesday	
Movement	Light 10 minutes of stretching at home
Nutrition	Have a protein-rich snack mid-morning
Beauty/ Skincare	Apply SPF 30+ before going outside
Mindset/ Stress Reduction	Practice three minutes of mindfulness
Sleep Support	Turn your phone off and remove it from the bedroom (you will need to get yourself an alarm clock)
Day: Thursday	
Movement	Include some strength training to help preserve muscle mass, support bone health
Nutrition	Add colourful fruit and veggies to your dinner plate
Beauty/ Skincare	Do a light facial massage to boost circulation or some face yoga
Mindset/ Stress Reduction	Take a short walk or step outside
Sleep Support	Reduce caffeine intake
Day: Friday	
Movement	Dance to your favourite song in the kitchen
Nutrition	Focus on a fibre-rich lunch and add a spoonful of flaxseeds to your breakfast
Beauty/ Skincare	Apply a hydrating serum or mask in the evening. You can use a night mask that you can

	leave on all night to save time
Mindset/ Stress Reduction	Reflect on a small win from the week Listen to a calming playlist in the evening
Extra	Plan a weekend treat or evening with your girlfriends
Day: Saturday	
Movement	Walk with a friend or family member
Nutrition	Make a smoothie with protein and healthy fats
Beauty/ Skincare	Relaxing bath with essential oils or Epsom salts
Mindset/ Stress Reduction	Disconnect from screens for 30 minutes
Sleep Support	Ensure a dark, cool sleeping environment
Day: Sunday	
Movement	Do some sort of strength training
Nutrition	Prepare balanced meals for the week ahead
Beauty/ Skincare	Use a facial roller for lymphatic drainage or Gua Sha comb for your scalp
Mindset/ Stress Reduction	Set your intentions for the coming week
Sleep Support	Drink a cup of lemon balm tea and relax an hour before bed

Moving forward through perimenopause, menopause and beyond

This wellness plan isn't just a list of to-dos; it's designed to grow with you. Whether you're going through perimenopause, menopause, or post menopause, these routines or the routines you choose to make are here to support you, they are not here to make you feel stressed or tied down. They're adaptable, evolving as your needs shift, creating a foundation that respects where you are now and where you're headed.

As we move to the final chapters, we'll look at how to carry these habits forward, shaping a lifestyle that brings more joy, strength and control into each day. Let this be your launchpad for a fulfilling, vibrant future in the next phase of your life that honours who you are and supports who you want to be.

For many women, the path to better health can feel like a mountain to climb especially with so much advice urging big leaps and drastic changes. But there's a simpler, kinder approach. By focusing on just a small, 1% improvement each day, you make progress feel achievable and less overwhelming. Think of it as building a foundation, slowly, without expecting an immediate overhaul. As the saying goes, "The journey of a thousand miles begins with a single step," and in this case, each step builds momentum, paving the way for real, lasting wellness.

Three Quick Wins

1. Keep a "low energy day" list on your fridge - so you're always prepared to do something even when you feel like doing nothing.

2. Choose a daily non-negotiable – something so small it's impossible to skip (like one deep breath before your morning coffee or applying a night cream before bed).

3. Write a One-Word Journal - each night, write one word that sums up your day. It builds awareness without pressure and helps track emotional patterns.

12 LIVING WELL IN THE LONG RUN: WHAT HAPPENS NEXT

"Every day is a new opportunity to change your life and be who you want to be."

Demi Lovato

Five Things You'll Learn in this Chapter:

- **How to create a personal wellness vision** that reflects your goals and values

- **The power of small daily choices** for long-term health and happiness

- **How to embrace ageing with confidence,** purpose and grace

- **Supportive** strategies to help you feel energised, balanced and strong

- Ideas for building your own **go-to health and beauty wellness kit.**

Envisioning the Life You Want to Live

As we move into the next exciting chapter of your life, it's natural to wonder what lies ahead. Your wellness and happiness are no longer just about getting through each day but about truly thriving and feeling vibrant and fulfilled. This isn't about just "keeping up" but about stepping into a version of yourself that feels grounded, comfortable with who you are, happy and inspired. So, take a moment to consider the life you envision for yourself. What does it look like? How do you want to feel, not just now but in the years ahead, through perimenopause, menopause and post-menopause?

Creating a Personal Wellness Vision

Imagine your future health, well-being and how you want to look and feel as you move through this stage of life. Think beyond routines or checklists; this is about painting a picture of your life in a way that excites you. Maybe you see yourself embracing new hobbies, spending time with loved ones, exploring travel, or doing activities that bring you joy. Perhaps you'd like to feel confident in your energy levels, comfortable in your body and proud of the way you look, have glowing skin, healthy hair, feel comfortable in your own body with a sense of vitality that reflects all the care you've invested in yourself. This vision of wellness isn't just about physical health but about mental and emotional fulfilment as well, embracing beauty from within that radiates outward.

The Role of HRT and Personal Choice

For some, hormone replacement therapy (HRT) might be part of this journey through menopause. If you've chosen HRT, it can be a valuable support, working alongside the nourishing lifestyle habits you're building. If HRT isn't your path, rest assured that natural approaches can be powerful. What's unique here is that whether or not you choose HRT, the practices in this book are designed to work for you. This journey is deeply personal and the choices you make about your body should always feel aligned with your own values, needs and comfort.

Action Step – Future Journal Exercise

To help bring this vision to life, try a brief journaling exercise. Grab a notebook and write a letter to your future self. Describe the life you want to lead and the feelings you wish to cultivate daily. What does a day in this future life of yours look like? How does your body feel? How are you spending your time and who are you sharing it with? This exercise isn't about perfection or rigid goals but about setting a foundation that's full of possibility and hope.

To give you an idea of how this letter might look, here's a letter I wrote to myself from my own perspective. As I wrote it, I reflected on my journey, finding natural solutions to support my wellness and balance without HRT. Take this as a gentle guide, then try your own version, letting your unique vision shape the words. Remember, this is a personal, hopeful message from you to you. It's the encouragement to embrace every possibility that comes with this next phase of your life.

Dear future me,

I hope this finds you in a place of health, happiness and balance, one you've worked so hard to achieve. I imagine you're feeling good in your body, confident in your choices and you have the kind of energy that comes from taking care of yourself in a way that feels right for you.

You've embraced this phase of life with a sense of curiosity and strength, figuring out what works for you without the pressure of perfection. Some days might still see challenging hormonal shifts, low energy and changes in how you look or feel but you've found ways to support yourself through it.

You've learnt to listen to your body. Whether it's starting the day with a moment of calm, prioritising nourishing meals, or taking a little extra time to care for your skin, these habits reflect your commitment to yourself. Even without HRT, you've found natural solutions that help you feel more balanced and in control.

You've created a life that feels good. A life where you wake up knowing you're capable of handling whatever comes your way. You've embraced the woman you are, with all her beauty, strength and imperfections and you've made her your priority.

Here's to the woman who didn't give up on herself. You've shown that small steps, done consistently, can create a life where you feel strong, beautiful and ready to take on whatever comes next.

Love

Alison

A Holistic Approach to Ageing Well

Now that you've created a personal vision for the life you want, let's look at supportive practices to bring that vision to life each day. Ageing well isn't about clinging to youth but about embracing the unique beauty, wisdom and strength of each stage, especially as we move through perimenopause, menopause and beyond. My approach here focuses on positive ageing, nurturing every part of your body, mind and spirit so that you thrive not only in how you look but in how you feel about yourself. After all, we all want to feel good in our own skin, to see a reflection that we like which feels vibrant, healthy and truly us.

For me, keeping mentally sharp is one of the most fulfilling parts of ageing well. Simple activities like puzzles, reading, or trying something new can keep the mind fresh and curious. I took up golf a few years ago during Covid and that has been a great way to keep my brain sharp! These moments aren't just about preventing brain fog; they're about discovering joy and purpose in each day. Staying connected to our interests and passions keeps us mentally strong.

"Your future self is built on the choices you make today. Start small, stay consistent and keep going."

ss

As for physical health, it's something I've come to value more deeply with each passing year. Hormonal changes can affect everything from skin texture to joint health, so it's important to find gentle, restorative ways to move. Exercises like yoga, stretching, or swimming that are easy on the joints keep us flexible, strong and energised. And skincare matters here too, choosing products that feel good, and hydrating helps us feel confident as our skin's needs evolve.

Then there's digestive health, often overlooked, but essential to feeling vibrant. As we age, easy-to-digest foods rich in nutrients can make all the difference in our energy and balance. I'm a big believer in adding more fibre, staying hydrated and focusing on meals that support your well-being from the inside out. When we feel good on the inside, it naturally shows, giving us a glow that reflects health and confidence.

With this holistic approach, we're nourishing every part of ourselves, body, mind and spirit, to support positive ageing but about feeling happy, beautiful and strong in the body and mind you have today. Embracing positive ageing means greeting each day with gratitude, knowing we're living in a body we can feel proud of and comfortable in at every stage of our journey.

As you map out this next phase of life, let it be an empowering reminder: wellness is a journey that evolves as you do. Embrace the freedom to shape this life on your terms, whether through HRT, lifestyle changes, beauty routines or a mix of them all. This is your time to thrive, to shape a fulfilling future that grows with you.

"Your body may be changing, but it's still yours. Treat it with the love, care and respect it deserves."

Alison Bladh

As we come to the end of this book, I'd love to help you create your own health and beauty wellness kit, a supportive collection of simple tools and ideas you can turn to when life feels bumpy. Think of this kit as your go-to wellness companion, something that brings calm, clarity and confidence, especially on tougher days.

The example kit below offers three core items in each area to get you started. These are your foundation, small things that make a big difference. As you go forward, you can personalise and build on your kit. Add the things that work for you, bring you comfort and help you feel your best.

> *"Ageing is not lost youth but a new stage of*
> *opportunity and strength."*
>
> **Betty Friedan**

Health and Beauty Wellness Kit

Nutrition

1. Protein Power Bowl Recipe – A go-to meal formula that includes greens, protein (like beans, eggs, or chicken), healthy fats (avocado, nuts), and a squeeze of lemon for flavour.

2. Anti-Inflammatory Spice Blend – Keep a jar of turmeric, ginger and black pepper mix to sprinkle on foods, helping reduce inflammation.

3. Digestive Bitters – Use before meals to support digestion and reduce bloating. A few drops of bitters on the tongue can aid in nutrient absorption, especially during menopause.

Movement

1. Desk-Friendly Stretch Routine – A short series of stretches that can be done at your desk to relieve tension in the neck, shoulders and back.

2. Balance Training – Practice standing on one leg while brushing your teeth or cooking, building core strength and stability.

3. Mini Resistance Bands – Keep these inexpensive bands handy for quick strength training that targets glutes, arms and core without taking up space.

Sleep

1. Sleepy Tea Blend – Drink a cup of chamomile, passionflower or valerian root tea about 60 minutes before bed to promote relaxation and improve sleep quality.

2. Lavender Pillow Spray – Spritz lavender essential oil mixed with distilled water onto your pillow for a calming effect that helps ease you into sleep.

3. Evening Blue Light Glasses – Use blue light blocking glasses in the evening to reduce eye strain and signal to your brain that it's time to wind down.

Skincare

1. Gua Sha Stone - A Gua sha stone, typically made of Jade or Bian stone (a mineral-rich black stone used in traditional Chinese medicine), can be gently massaged along the face to promote lymphatic drainage, reduce puffiness, and improve skin elasticity. It's a simple tool that adds a revitalising step to your skincare routine.

2. Hydrating Face Mist – Choose a hydrating face mist with cooling ingredients. Not only does it provide a quick, refreshing boost for your skin, but it's also perfect for soothing hot flushes and helping you feel revitalised throughout the day.

3. Vitamin C Serum – Use in the morning to boost skin's brightness and protect against environmental stressors.

Mental clarity

1. Brain-Boosting Nootropic Teas – Teas like ginkgo biloba, rosemary and green tea to support focus and mental clarity.

2. 5-Minute Brain Dump – Keep a notebook by your bedside to jot down thoughts and ideas at the end of the day, clearing your mind for better focus and restful sleep.

3. Brain Fog Buster Breathing Exercise – Practice a simple, energising breathing technique like "box breathing." Inhale for 4 counts, hold for 4, exhale for 4 and pause for 4. This quick exercise can help clear mental fog, bringing clarity and focus.

Stress relief

1. Pocket Aromatherapy Oil – Keep a small bottle of calming essential oils like lavender, frankincense or bergamot in your handbag. When you need a moment of calm, simply place a drop on a tissue and inhale deeply. This quick, on-the-go solution brings instant relaxation and helps ease stress wherever you are. You can also have the oil on a tissue and keep it in your bra. Here you can smell it by gently taking it out and sniffing it when needed.

2. Grounding Mat – Use a grounding mat for a few minutes each day to reduce stress and boost mood, especially useful for menopause-related anxiety.

3. Mini Acupressure Tool - A small acupressure ring or handheld tool can help stimulate relaxation points on your fingers or hands, offering quick tension relief.

4. Noise-Cancelling Earbuds - Escape into a calming playlist, white noise, or a guided meditation to create a peaceful moment, even in a noisy environment.

Hormone balancing

1. Phytoestrogen-Rich Foods – Incorporate foods like flaxseeds, chickpeas and soy products, which contain plant-based compounds that have a similar chemical structure to oestrogen. These phytoestrogens may help alleviate hot flushes, night sweats and mood changes, providing gentle, natural support during hormonal transitions.

2. Liver-Supportive Herbs (Milk Thistle & Dandelion) – The liver plays a crucial role in hormone processing and detoxification. Milk thistle and dandelion root are gentle, supportive herbs that can help the liver metabolise hormones more effectively. A liver-supportive herbal tea may help with balancing hormones and managing symptoms like skin changes and fatigue.

3. Portable Snack Packs – Keep pre-packaged, hormone-friendly snacks like nuts, seeds, boiled eggs and protein rich snacks on hand. These balanced snacks help stabilise blood sugar, support energy and make it easy to nourish yourself on busy days.

"Wellness isn't a destination, it's a lifelong journey of small, intentional choices. The way you care for yourself today shapes the energy, confidence and vitality you'll carry into the years ahead."

Alison Bladh

As we come to the end of this chapter, remember that this book is here as your companion offering guidance, encouragement, and practical support as you move forward, think of this book as your trusted companion, something you can return to again and again whenever you need a boost, a reminder or a little encouragement. Life will continue to bring changes and challenges, but now you have a toolkit of practical strategies, nourishing insights and realistic ideas to support you through every stage of perimenopause, menopause and postmenopause.

This journey was never about perfection. It's about showing up for yourself with patience, presence and self-compassion. Each section in this book offers flexible resources that can meet you wherever you are. Use what speaks to you, revisit what works and allow your approach to evolve as you do.

Keep this book close, your no-nonsense guide to looking and feeling good, inside and out. Here's to a life of wellness that reflects your strength, honours your needs and celebrates who you truly are.

My tips for a happy life. What I do...

- I laugh daily even when things are feeling bad. Laughter has saved me many times throughout my life as I have always been able to see the funny side of things! Well, most things!
- I spend time with my family and friends
- I don't shy away from telling people I love them
- I do things that make me smile
- I let myself be ok with wanting to look good -it's not vain!
- I'm not afraid to say no
- I buy a new handbag at least once a year!
- I cry when I need to
- I feel ok with wanting to look my best
- I body brush everyday
- I use an Infrared sauna twice a week
- I go cold water bathing in a frozen lake!
- I have a facial once a month
- I will try anything once - if I don't like it I don't have to do it again.
- I have no regrets - I learn from my mistakes
- I do things that push me, even if they feel scary!
- I try to have a positive outlook on life
- I don't give up even when things get tough
- I choose to nourish my body with wholesome non-processed foods.

Three Quick Wins

1. Write a Letter to Your Future Self – Take five minutes to jot down how you want to feel and live in the years ahead. Keep it positive, encouraging and personal.

2. Create a Mini Wellness Kit – Choose one item from each area (nutrition, movement, skincare, stress, mindset) and keep them visible as daily reminders.

3. Set a Weekly Joy Goal – Pick one small thing each week that brings you joy—like a walk in nature, a face mask, or time with a friend—and schedule it in like an appointment.

13 WHAT I WISH I'D KNOWN ABOUT MENOPAUSE AT 30: TIPS FOR PREPARING YOUR BODY AND MIND FOR A SMOOTHER TRANSITION

"The habits you build in your 30s shape the woman you'll be in your 50s. Start now – your future self will thank you."

Alison Bladh

Five Things You'll Learn in this Chapter:

- **Why your 30s and 40s matter** – How your daily habits now shape the ease of your perimenopause and menopause journey later.

- **What no one told you** – The real signs and symptoms of menopause that often catch women off guard.

- **How to future-proof your body and mind** – From blood sugar balance to bone support, discover practical prevention strategies.

- **Why skin, sleep and stress deserve attention early** – Small actions now can dramatically impact how you look and feel later.

- **That menopause isn't the end, it's a new beginning** – With the right prep, it can be an empowering, freeing stage of life.

If I could go back and have a chat with my 30-year-old self, I'd have a lot to say and that's exactly why I wrote this bonus chapter. I knew this book wouldn't be complete without it. Because the truth is, everything we do in our 30s can shape the way we move through perimenopause, menopause and postmenopause and I wish I'd understood that earlier.

At 30, I thought menopause was something that happened to older women, far in the future. I was busy living life, chasing dreams and thinking about everything but my hormones. No one was talking about this stage of life in any real or relatable way. But now, after years of working with women and going through it myself, I know that menopause isn't just a moment in time, it's a journey built on everything that's come before.

This chapter is here to share what I wish someone had told me. That menopause isn't a sudden switch, but a gradual recalibration of your body, your mind and how you see yourself. That our stress, sleep, eating habits and even how we speak to ourselves all play a part. This isn't about fear or blame, it's about knowledge, confidence and feeling prepared.

In many cultures, menopausal women are revered as wise leaders and heads of their communities, a perspective often linked to fewer symptoms and a smoother transition than women in the Western world.

And let me be real here, menopause can be shit! Many women will nod in agreement at that and rightly so. The sleepless nights, the hot flushes, the relentless brain fog, and the emotional rollercoaster can make you feel like you're losing your mind and grip. But here's the thing: it doesn't last forever. When you come out the other side, there's a freedom waiting for you that's unlike anything else. A freedom where you don't really care what anyone else thinks of you is so powerful and liberating!

58% of women under the age of 40 say they don't feel at all informed about menopause.

"One of the best things about getting older? You stop giving a damn about the nonsense. Your tolerance for drama shrinks, your love for comfort grows and suddenly, 'no' becomes your favourite word."

Alison Bladh

I can tell you, once the storm settles, menopause can be truly liberating. You stop caring about what people think, and you start living for yourself. You develop a sense of unapologetic confidence, where you feel deeply grounded in yourself and embrace the freedom to live life on your terms. That's the part no one tells you, the strength and clarity that come after the chaos.

"At this age, I wear what I like, say what I think and do what makes me happy because frankly, I've run out of patience for anything else."

Alison Bladh

So, here's what I wish I'd known at 30: Menopause is not the enemy. It's a natural transition and while it comes with its challenges, it also comes with power. The power to know yourself better, to prioritise what really matters and to reclaim your energy and health in ways you never thought possible.

This chapter isn't just for those of us who've crossed that threshold. It's for 30-year-old me (and you) and for every woman in her 20s, 30s, or 40s who hasn't quite reached menopause but wants to feel prepared, not blindsided. It's a guide to understanding what you can do now to build the foundation for a healthier, stronger, and more vibrant future.

Let's have a look into the wisdom I wish I'd had back then; the things I want every younger woman to know. Because while we can't turn back the clock, we can pass on the lessons and make sure the next generation has the knowledge and tools to embrace this chapter of life with confidence and understanding.

"I don't think we talk about menopause enough. It's like a shush-shush topic. But it shouldn't be. Women need to know what's happening to their bodies."

Michelle Obama

Things I Wish I'd Known About Menopause at 30

Menopause Can Be Messy and That's Okay

No one tells you that menopause isn't just hot flushes and mood swings. It can be unpredictable, overwhelming and downright exhausting. Knowing this in advance can help you approach it with more understanding and less frustration. And yes, some days, it can feel utterly shit. But acknowledging that it's normal makes it easier to navigate.

It's Not Just About Periods Stopping

Menopause affects everything from your energy levels and sleep to your skin, joints and even your digestion. It's a whole-body experience, not just a reproductive one, and that's why understanding it early is so important. The decline in oestrogen and progesterone affects nearly every bodily system!

Your body will demand you listen

You can't push through menopause like you might have with other challenges in life. Your body will insist that you slow down, rest and take better care of yourself or it will force you to. Learning to listen to your body now will serve you well later. You might think you can carry on with the late nights and boozy weekends, but I can assure you, you can't! I speak from experience.

Weight Redistribution Happens Even If You Don't Gain Weight

Your shape might change even if the scales don't. Fat tends to settle around your middle, which can feel frustrating. But it's not a reflection of failure, it's your body adapting to hormonal shifts. You could go from a pear shape to an apple shape.

Hormones are powerful and complex

Oestrogen, progesterone and testosterone aren't just about reproduction. They influence your mood, memory, energy, looks and even your confidence. Understanding this earlier would have made the roller coaster so much easier to handle.

It Can Mess with Your Head

Brain fog, forgetfulness and emotional ups and downs are real. It's like your brain suddenly feels scrambled. Knowing this is part of the process would have been a huge relief at the time.

Protect and Preserve: Beauty Tips for Ageing Gracefully

Taking care of your skin in your 30s and 40s lays the foundation for looking and feeling your best as you age. Sun exposure, lifestyle habits and hormonal shifts can all impact your skin's health, but taking pre-emptive steps now can make a world of difference.

Wear sunscreen 30+ daily to protect against UV damage, prioritise hydration with moisturisers and plenty of water and include collagen-boosting foods like salmon and citrus in your diet. At night, cleanse gently, apply nourishing serum and creams that suits your skin type and finish with a nourishing eye cream and neck cream if you really want to look after yourself.

Alcohol and Hormones: A Recipe for Discomfort

You might not relate to this now, but I can promise you, you will when you're in it. Alcohol tends to amplify menopausal symptoms like hot flushes, poor sleep and mood swings. What used to be a harmless glass of wine might suddenly feel like a full-on attack on your system. Start experimenting with reducing alcohol or finding alternatives that you enjoy, like herbal teas or sparkling water with fresh fruit. You'll thank yourself later.

You Don't Have to Suffer in Silence

There's so much help available - HRT, supplements, nutritional therapy, lifestyle tweaks that can make a massive difference. The hardest part is asking for help, but once you do, it opens the door to solutions.

Self-Care Is Non-Negotiable

The days of putting yourself last need to end. Self-care isn't indulgent it's essential. Learning to prioritise yourself now will make the transition through menopause so much smoother.

Menopause can be Empowering

It's not all doom and gloom. On the other side, many women feel freer, more confident and less inclined to care about what others think. It's a time to rediscover and redefine yourself.

Your Skin and Hair Need New Attention

As hormone levels drop, your old skincare and haircare routines might not work like they used to. Adapting to these changes can help you feel more confident about how you look.

Community is Everything

Connecting with other women going through the same thing is invaluable. Shared experiences and advice make the journey feel less isolating. Find your tribe.

It's Never Too Early to Prepare

What you do in your 30s and 40s like eating well, managing stress, looking after your skin and exercising can set you up for a smoother menopause transition. Start building those habits now.

Support your Bones with Vitamin D and Vitamin K

Bone health becomes increasingly important as oestrogen declines, making Vitamin D and K essential. Vitamin D helps your body absorb calcium, while Vitamin K ensures that calcium goes to your bones where it's needed, rather than your arteries. Studies show that women who looked after their bones before perimenopause had a lower risk of developing osteopenia and osteoporosis in later life.

Action Point: Include foods rich in these vitamins, like fatty fish, green leafy vegetables and eggs. Consider supplements if needed, especially during winter months.

You're Not Alone in Feeling Lost

So many women feel blindsided by menopause because no one talks about it enough. Knowing you're not alone can be comforting.

Your Libido Might Change

Sexual health is another area affected by menopause, but it's manageable. Open conversations and finding solutions that work for you can make all the difference.

Menopause Isn't the End - It's A New Beginning

Yes, menopause is challenging, but it's also an invitation to step into a new chapter with greater wisdom, deeper confidence and a freedom you've never felt before. Embrace the journey and don't regret getting older as it's a privilege denied to many.

"Menopause isn't a cliff we fall off, it's a transition we walk through and how we prepare for it makes all the difference."

Alison Bladh

What You Can Do Now:
16 Smart Strategies for a Smoother Transition Later

Menopause doesn't start the day your periods stop, it's a journey built on years of choices, habits and how well you've cared for yourself leading up to it. The good news? There's so much you can do in your 30s and 40s to support your body and mind before the hormonal shifts begin.

Knowledge is key. Once you understand what's going on inside your body, you're in a far better place to decide how you want to support it whether through lifestyle changes, medical options, or a personalised mix that works for you. These practical, prevention-focused steps are the ones I wish I'd started earlier and they can make all the difference to how you feel when menopause arrives.

1. Build Muscle Now

Why It Matters: As women age, muscle mass naturally declines and this can slow metabolism and contribute to weight gain during menopause. Building muscle in your 30s and 40s lays the foundation for a stronger, leaner body later.

What to Do: Incorporate strength training 2-3 times a week. It's not just all about aesthetics; strong muscles support healthy bones and improve metabolic health, both crucial during menopause.

2. Prioritise Gut Health

Why It Matters: A healthy gut helps metabolise hormones, manage weight and regulate mood. Gut issues can amplify menopausal symptoms like bloating, fatigue, and even anxiety.

What to Do: Start eating a diverse range of plant-based foods now. Aim for 30 different plants a week, including fruits, vegetables, nuts, seeds and whole grains. Add fermented foods like kefir or kimchi to support gut diversity.

3. Support your Bones

Why It Matters: Oestrogen plays a critical role in maintaining bone density. As levels decline in menopause, women are at higher risk of osteoporosis. Laying the groundwork for strong bones starts well before menopause.

What to Do: Incorporate calcium-rich foods like leafy greens, almonds and dairy. Ensure you're getting vitamin D from sunshine or supplements and do weight-bearing exercises.

4. Manage Stress Proactively

Why It Matters: High cortisol levels can disrupt hormone balance, affect sleep and lead to weight gain. Chronic stress can make menopause symptoms like hot flushes and brain fog worse.

What to Do: Develop stress-relief habits now, such as mindfulness, yoga, or journaling. Small, consistent practices can build resilience for the more hormonal shifts to come.

5. Protect and Preserve: Beauty Tips for Ageing Gracefully

Why It Matters: Skin ageing starts earlier than many of us think and how you care for your skin in your 30s and 40s can make a big difference later. Hormonal changes, sun exposure and lifestyle habits all affect skin health but taking action now can help maintain elasticity, hydration and that radiant glow well into your later years.

What to Do: Wear SPF daily to protect against UV damage, hydrate with moisturisers and plenty of water, and nourish your skin from within by eating foods rich in vitamin C, zinc and collagen (like salmon, citrus and leafy greens). You might also consider a high-quality collagen supplement. At night, cleanse gently, apply a serum and finish with a nourishing cream to support skin repair while you sleep.

6. Focus on Sleep Hygiene

Why it Matters: Sleep quality often declines during menopause due to night sweats, hormonal changes and anxiety. Poor sleep can impact weight, mood and overall health considerably

What to Do: Create a bedtime routine that promotes relaxation. Dim lights an hour before bed, avoid screens and drink calming teas like chamomile. The better your sleep hygiene now, the easier it will be to adapt when your hormones fluctuate.

7. Balance your Blood Sugar

Why it Matters: Blood sugar imbalances can lead to insulin resistance, weight gain, and fatigue all of which become harder to manage during menopause.

What to Do: Start eating balanced meals with protein, healthy fats and fibre. Avoid ultra processed foods, sugary snacks and refined carbs. Building this habit early will help regulate energy levels and curb cravings later in life.

8. Understand your Hormones

Why It Matters: Hormonal changes don't just appear overnight they often begin with subtle shifts in mood, energy, skin or sleep. Understanding how hormones like oestrogen, progesterone and testosterone work and tracking your cycle, can help you notice changes early and take proactive steps.

What to Do: Use a period tracking app or notebook to log physical and emotional symptoms. If you notice irregularities, speak to a healthcare professional. Awareness is empowering it helps you respond with confidence rather than react with confusion.

9. Strengthen Your Emotional Health

Why It Matters: Emotional well-being plays a significant role in how you navigate menopause. Feeling grounded and confident makes it easier to handle symptoms and changes.

What to Do: Start building self-care habits and exploring what makes you feel good. This could be as simple as taking time for a hobby, talking to a therapist, or setting boundaries like learning to say no.

10. Build a Lifestyle you Love

Why it Matters: The habits you form in your younger years often dictate how you approach health and wellness later. A sedentary, high-stress lifestyle will only make menopause more challenging.

What to Do: Take stock of your daily habits. Are you moving enough, eating nourishing foods, and prioritising rest? Small, consistent changes now can have an impact later.

11. Educate Yourself

Why it Matters: Many women enter menopause with no idea what's happening to their bodies. Knowledge is empowering and allows you to prepare emotionally and physically for the transition.

What to Do: Read books, listen to podcasts and follow credible experts. Seek out community support groups or friends willing to share their experiences to reduce the stigma and fear surrounding menopause.

12. Strengthen Your Pelvic Floor

Why It Matters: Oestrogen decline can weaken pelvic floor muscles, leading to bladder issues and affecting sexual wellness. Strengthening them early offers long-term protection.

What to Do: Practise daily pelvic floor exercises like Kegels or try Pilates-based movement that targets the core. Even just a few minutes a day can make a big difference.

13. Nourish with Healthy Fats

Why It Matters: Healthy fats are vital for hormone production, skin health and brain function all of which become more important as we age.

What to Do: Include foods like avocado, nuts, olive oil, flaxseed and oily fish in your meals regularly. These fats support mood, hormones and skin health. Focus on foods rich in vitamin C, zinc and collagen. Consider adding a high-quality collagen supplement if needed and don't forget daily SPF.

14. Build Your Inner Circle of Support

Why It Matters: Women who feel supported emotionally tend to cope better with menopause. Connection helps reduce stress and builds emotional resilience.

What to Do: Invest in relationships that nourish you. Make time for friends who listen, laugh and lift you up. Join a group or start one because connection is medicine.

15. Rethink Alcohol and Caffeine Now

Why It Matters: While not "bad" per se, alcohol and caffeine can have a heightened impact on hormonal health, sleep, anxiety and skin as you age. Many women find these become less well-tolerated during perimenopause.

What to Do: Start paying attention to how you feel after your second coffee or evening glass of wine. Begin reducing intake or swapping in alternatives like herbal teas, chicory coffee or mocktails, so it's easier to adjust when your body becomes more sensitive.

16. Get Comfortable with Boundaries

Why It Matters: People-pleasing and overextending yourself becomes deeply exhausting as you age. Setting boundaries protects your energy, which becomes even more precious during hormonal shifts. Emotional health plays a huge role in menopause resilience.

What to Do: Practice saying "no" with kindness, delegate more often and identify the emotional triggers that deplete you. Journaling, therapy, or coaching in your 30s can build emotional tools you'll lean on for life.

Three Quick Wins
(Your Future Self Will Thank You For)

1. Start Resistance Training – Your Way

Begin strength training in a way that suits your lifestyle, no gym required. Use resistance bands at home, try a bodyweight workout online, or do squats while the kettle boils. What matters is getting started.

2. Cut Back on Ultra-Processed Foods

Reduce or avoid ultra-processed snacks and meals that spike your blood sugar. Choose whole, nourishing foods that fuel your hormones and support steady energy.

3. Find a Go-To Stress Tool

Pick one calming practice you can use daily to manage stress whether it's deep breathing, journaling, or a mindful walk. A few minutes a day can make a big difference to your hormone balance.

POEM

I want to leave you with the beautiful words of María Sabina, a Mexican healer and poet. Her wisdom is a powerful reminder that true healing often begins with nature, stillness and the simple things that nourish us.

"Heal yourself with the light of the sun and the rays of the moon.
With the sound of the river and the waterfall.
With the swaying of the sea and the fluttering of birds.
Heal yourself with mint, neem and eucalyptus.
Sweeten with lavender, rosemary and chamomile.
Hug yourself with the cocoa bean and a hint of cinnamon.
Put love in tea instead of sugar and drink it looking at the stars.
Heal yourself with the kisses that the wind gives you and the hugs of the rain.
Stand strong with your bare feet on the ground and with everything that comes from it.
Be smarter every day by listening to your intuition, looking at the world with your forehead.
Jump, dance, sing, so that you live happier.
Heal yourself, with beautiful love and always remember…
You are the medicine."

Attributed to María Sabina
(Mexican healer and poet)

ABOUT THE AUTHOR

Alison Bladh is an award-winning nutritional therapist and beauty therapist with over 35 years of experience specialising in women's health, particularly during perimenopause, menopause and beyond. As a registered professional, Alison is passionate about empowering women to not only feel good but also look their best.

With a unique background combining beauty therapy and nutritional therapy, Alison's approach bridges the gap between looking good and feeling great. Her work has helped countless women regain their health improve their skin and navigate life's changes with practical, no-nonsense strategies.

Her unique approach combines practical, evidence-based advice with her deep understanding of how inner health and outer beauty work together. Unable to take hormone replacement therapy (HRT) herself, Alison has explored natural, realistic strategies that work for busy, overwhelmed women.

Beyond her professional expertise, Alison is a lover of the great outdoors, a keen golfer, hiker, scuba diver and even a beekeeper. She believes wellness should be simple, achievable and enjoyable because life's too short to chase perfection.

Alison's mission is simple: to help women take back control of their bodies, rediscover their energy and feel confident in their own skin without complicated routines or unrealistic expectations. She knows that menopause isn't the end of feeling amazing; it's a new beginning. Because looking good isn't just about vanity, it's about identity. It's about catching your reflection and recognising the woman staring back at you the one who feels strong, radiant and alive. This book is her gift to every woman who has ever looked in the mirror and wondered where she went. It's time to find her again!

WORK WITH ME

You've reached the end of the book but this is really just the beginning of your next chapter. Knowledge is powerful, but true transformation happens when you take action.

If you're ready to put what you've learned into practice with expert support, I'd love to guide you. I offer a range of programmes created specifically for women 40+ navigating perimenopause, menopause or post-menopause designed to help you boost energy, balance hormones, manage weight and feel confident in your body again. Read on to see how we can work together.

Ways We Can Work Together:

Join My 21-Day Body Reboot and Reset – A structured programme to increase energy, improve focus, and support sustainable weight loss through realistic nutrition, lifestyle, and mindset shifts. Scan QR code to learn more:

1:1 Nutritional therapy and lifestyle medicine – Personalised support tailored to your health goals, whether it's weight management, skincare, low energy, or hormonal balance. Let's build a plan that works for your life.

Book a Free Discovery Call – Not sure what's right for you? Let's talk. This free chat will help you get clear on your next step.

Ready to Start?

You don't have to do this alone. My programmes are designed to be simple, effective and achievable even in a busy life. Because real change should feel empowering, not overwhelming.

Visit *www.alisonbladh.com* to explore programmes and book your place:

Questions? Email me at contact@alisonbladh.com

You've done the reading now let's turn it into action so you can feel like yourself again: energised, balanced and back in control.

YOUR WELLNESS PROMISE PLANNER

This planner is your space to turn small changes into long-term habits. It's simple, doable and designed to help you stay on track with what matters most. Download it using the QR code below to access a digital version, or you can fill it in directly in the book.

My Wellness Commitment

Over the next 12 weeks, I'm committing to one small, positive change each month that supports my health and wellbeing. By writing down my goals, I'll stay focused, motivated and accountable because real progress is built on consistency, not perfection.

Wellness Commitment Card

Your Personal Wellness Promise

Name: _____

Start Date: _____

My Wellness Commitment:

Reflecting on what I've learned, I commit to making a small, positive change each month over the next 12 weeks. Writing down my goals will help me stay accountable and stick to them.

Change I Will Make and Stick To:

Month 1: _____

Month 2: _____

Month 3: _____

Why These Changes Matter to Me:

_____

_____

_____

_____

Remember:

- One change at a time, each month small steps can add up to big improvements in how you feel and look.

- Writing it down helps make your goals feel real and reachable.

- Stay connected, share your progress with friends or community for motivation and support.

Daily Wellness Log

Day	Wellness Focus	Movement	Nutrition	Skincare	Mindfulness & Self Care	Reflection
Monday						
Tuesday						
Wednesday						
Thursday						
Friday						
Saturday						
Sunday						

Using Your Planner

Wellness Focus: Set a simple goal for each day, such as stress management, energy or hydration to stay focused on one aspect of wellness.

Movement: Choose any form of movement that feels achievable. Include gentle stretches, short walks, or even a quick dance in the kitchen.

Nutrition: Pick one nutrition goal, like adding a vegetable serving, drinking a extra glass of water, or reducing sugar.

Skincare: Add a self-care step to your skincare routine. This could be something like applying SPF, using a gentle exfoliant, or taking five minutes for a face mask.

Mindfulness & Self-Care: This section is for simple mindfulness moments or relaxation exercises, like a breathing exercise before bed or setting intentions in the morning.

Reflection: Use the end-of-day reflection to capture your thoughts and celebrate any progress. What felt good? What small wins did you notice?

This planner helps you keep wellness balanced and adaptable to your own needs, encouraging a gentle, daily commitment to overall well-being.

RESOURCES

These websites, books and apps can help support your health, wellbeing and menopause journey. They offer trustworthy advice, tools, and guidance when you want to learn more, track symptoms, or explore further support.

Menopause & Hormone Health

- North American Menopause Society (NAMS) – https://menopause.org
- National Institute on Aging (NIA) – https://www.nia.nih.gov
- British Menopause Society – https://thebms.org.uk
- Women's Health Concern – https://www.womens-health-concern.org
- NICE Guidelines – https://www.nice.org.uk
- Newson Health – https://www.newsonhealth.co.uk
- European Menopause and Andropause Society (EMAS) https://emas-online.org/
- Balance App for Menopause Support – https://www.balance-menopause.com/balance-app
- A4M – The American Academy of Anti-Aging Medicine – https://www.a4m.com

Premature Ovarian Insufficiency (POI)

- Daisy Network – POI Charity – https://www.daisynetwork.org

Nutrition & Functional Medicine

- Institute for Functional Medicine – https://www.ifm.orgBritish Association for Nutrition and Lifestyle Medicine (BANT) – https://bant.org.uk
- Dirty Dozen & Clean 15 Guide – https://www.ewg.org/foodnews/clean-fifteen.php
- Blood sugar monitor - https://www.hellolingo.com/uk

Period and Symptom Tracking

- Flo Period Tracker App – https://flo.health
- Balance Menopause App – https://www.balance-menopause.com/balance-app

Sleep & Stress Support

- Calm App – https://www.calm.com
- Sleepio App – https://www.sleepio.com
- Headspace App – https://www.headspace.com
- The Sleep Foundation– https://www.sleepfoundation.org

Mental & Emotional Wellbeing

Mind (UK Mental Health Charity) – https://www.mind.org.uk

Beauty & Skincare

- CIDESCO – Comité International d'Esthétique et de Cosmétologie - https://cidesco.com
- SHR – Sveriges Hudterapeuters Riksorganisation - https://www.shr.nu

Heart Health

- British Heart Foundation – https://www.bhf.org.uk

Cold Therapy

- Wim Hof Method (Cold Therapy & Breathing) – https://www.wimhof.com

Women's Health & Intimate Care

- FemmePharma – https://www.femmepharma.com

Pelvic Floor Health

- Squeezy App – NHS-approved app to support pelvic floor exercises. https://www.squeezyapp.com/

Recipes & Nutrition Inspiration

- Alison Bladh Blog Recipes –
  https://www.alisonbladh.com/post?category=Recipes
- Alison Bladh Website – https://www.alisonbladh.com

Recommended Reading

- Atomic Habits by James Clear
- Oestrogen Matters by Dr Avrum Bluming and Dr Carol Tavris
- Fast Like a Girl by Dr Mindy Pelz

REFERENCES

Chapter 1

1. Croft, D.P., Brent, L.J.N., Franks, D.W. and Cant, M.A., 2017. Reproductive conflict and the evolution of menopause in killer whales. Current Biology, 27(2), pp.298–304.

2. Erdélyi, A., Pálfi, E., Tűű, L., Nas, K., Szűcs, Z., Török, M., Jakab, A. and Várbíró, S., 2023. The importance of nutrition in menopause and perimenopause: a review. Nutrients, 16(1), p.27. https://doi.org/10.3390/nu16010027

3. Fang, Y., Liu, F., Zhang, X., et al., 2024. Mapping global prevalence of menopausal symptoms among middle-aged women: a systematic review and meta-analysis. BMC Public Health, 24, p.1767. https://doi.org/10.1186/s12889-024-19280-5

4. Foster, E.A., Franks, D.W., Mazzi, S., et al., 2012. Adaptive prolonged postreproductive life span in killer whales. Science, 337, p.1313. DOI: 10.1126/science.1224198

5. Hawkes, K., O'Connell, J.F. and Blurton Jones, N.G., 1997. Hadza women's time allocation, offspring provisioning, and the evolution of long postmenopausal life spans. Current Anthropology, 38(4), pp.551–577.

6. Islam RM, Bell RJ, Green S, Page MJ, Davis SR. Safety and efficacy of testosterone for women: a systematic review and

meta-analysis of randomised controlled trial data. Lancet Diabetes Endocrinol. 2019 Oct;7(10):754-766. doi: 10.1016/S2213-8587(19)30189-5. Epub 2019 Jul 25. PMID: 31353194.

7. Karlamangla, A.S., Lachman, M.E., Han, W., Huang, M. and Greendale, G.A., 2017. Evidence for cognitive aging in midlife women: Study of Women's Health Across the Nation. PLoS ONE, 12(1), e0169008. https://doi.org/10.1371/journal.pone.0169008

8. Lambrinoudaki, I., Armeni, E., Goulis, D., Bretz, S., Ceausu, I., Durmusoglu, F., Erkkola, R., Fistonic, I., Gambacciani, M., Geukes, M., Hamoda, H., Hartley, C., Hirschberg, A.L., Meczekalski, B., Mendoza, N., Mueck, A., Smetnik, A., Stute, P., van Trotsenburg, M. and Rees, M., 2022. Menopause, wellbeing and health: A care pathway from the European Menopause and Andropause Society. Maturitas, 163, pp.1–14. https://doi.org/10.1016/j.maturitas.2022.04.008

9. McCarthy, M. and Raval, A.P., 2020. The peri-menopause in a woman's life: a systemic inflammatory phase that enables later neurodegenerative disease. Journal of Neuroinflammation, 17, p.317. https://doi.org/10.1186/s12974-020-01998-9

10. Moore, A., 2019. The French elaboration of ideas about menopause, sexuality and ageing. ResearchGate. https://www.researchgate.net/publication/335259685_The_Fr ench_Elaboration_of_Ideas_about_Menopause_Sexuality_and_ Ageing

11. Musial, N., Ali, Z., Grbevski, J., Veerakumar, A. and Sharma,

P., 2021. Perimenopause and first-onset mood disorders: a closer look. Focus (American Psychiatric Publishing), 19(3), pp.330–337. https://doi.org/10.1176/appi.focus.20200041

12. Nappi, R.E. and Cucinella, L., 2020. Long-term consequences of menopause. In: F. Petraglia and B. Fauser, eds. Female Reproductive Dysfunction. Cham: Springer. https://doi.org/10.1007/978-3-030-03594-5_17-1

13. National Institute for Health and Care Excellence (NICE), 2024. Menopause: identification and management [NG23]. London: NICE. Available at: https://www.nice.org.uk/guidance/ng23

14. Pope, A. and Wurlitzer, S., 2017. Wild power: discover the magic of your menstrual cycle and awaken the feminine path to power. London: Hay House.

15. Rzepecki, A.K., 2022. Updated perspectives on the role of estrogens in skin aging. Clinical, Cosmetic and Investigational Dermatology, 15, pp.1097–1108. https://doi.org/10.2147/CCID.S284123

16. Skae, F., 1865. Climacteric insanity. Edinburgh Medical Journal, 10(8), pp.703–716. PMID: 29646531; PMCID: PMC5308948.

17. Stachenfeld, N.S., Leone, C.A., Mitchell, E.S., Freese, E. and Harkness, L., 2018. Water intake reverses dehydration-associated impaired executive function in healthy young women. Physiology & Behavior, 185, pp.103–111. https://doi.org/10.1016/j.physbeh.2017.12.028

18. Statista, 2024. Menopause in Europe. [online] Available at: https://www.statista.com/topics/10558/menopause-in-

europe/#topicOverview

19. The British Menopause Society (BMS), 2023. National Survey Results: January 2023. [online] Available at: https://thebms.org.uk/wp-content/uploads/2023/01/BMS-Infographics-JANUARY-2023-NationalSurveyResults.pdf

20. Thornton, M.J., 2013. Estrogens and aging skin. Dermato-Endocrinology, 5(2), pp.264–270. https://doi.org/10.4161/derm.23872

21. World Health Organization (WHO), 2024. Menopause: fact sheet. [online] Available at: https://www.who.int/news-room/fact-sheets/detail/menopause

22. Yelland, S., Steenson, S., Creedon, A. and Stanner, S., 2023. The role of diet in managing menopausal symptoms: a narrative review. Nutrition Bulletin, 48(1), pp.43–65. https://doi.org/10.1111/nbu.12607

23. Xin, M.Q.L. and Lane, R., 2025. Exploring the clinical, psychological, and social relevance of menopause for trans and gender diverse people: a qualitative study. Menopause, 32(4), pp.288–294. https://pubmed.ncbi.nlm.nih.gov/39874451/

Chapter 2

1. American College of Obstetricians and Gynecologists, 2023. Mood Changes During Perimenopause Are Real. Here's What to Know. [online] Available at: https://www.acog.org/womens-health/experts-and-stories/the-latest/mood-changes-during-perimenopause-are-real-heres-what-to-know [Accessed 2 April 2025].

2. Crawford, S.L., Crandall, C.J., Derby, C.A., El Khoudary, S.R., Waetjen, L.E. and Avis, N.E., 2024. Use of vaginal estrogen and risk of breast cancer recurrence in survivors: A systematic review and meta-analysis. Menopause, 31(1), pp.15–24. doi:10.1097/GME.0000000000002105.

3. Duralde, E.R., Sobel, T.H. and Manson, J.E., 2023. Management of perimenopausal and menopausal symptoms. BMJ, 382, p.e072612. https://doi.org/10.1136/bmj-2022-072612

4. NHS, 2022. Menopause – Things you can do. [online] Available at: https://www.nhs.uk/conditions/menopause/things-you-can-do/ [Accessed 2 April 2025].

5. Panhandle Obstetrics and Gynecology, 2024. How Lifestyle Modifications Can Ease Your Menopausal Symptoms. [online] Available at: https://www.panhandleobgyn.com/post/how-lifestyle-modifications-can-ease-your-menopausal-symptoms [Accessed 2 April 2025].

6. Qian, J., Sun, S., Wang, M., Sun, Y., Sun, X., Jevitt, C. and Yu, X., 2023. The effect of exercise intervention on improving sleep in menopausal women: a systematic review and meta-analysis. Frontiers in Medicine, 10, p.1092294. https://doi.org/10.3389/fmed.2023.1092294

7. O'Connell, R.L., Risius, L., Slade, D., Smith, I.E., Bliss, J.M. and Loi, S., 2021. Hormone replacement therapy after breast cancer: A comprehensive review of safety and

recommendations. The Lancet Oncology, 22(11), pp.e456–
e467. doi:10.1016/S1470-2045(21)00451-2.

8. Schoenaker, D.A., Jackson, C.A., Rowlands, J.V. and Mishra,
G.D., 2014. Socioeconomic position, lifestyle factors and age
at natural menopause: a systematic review and meta-analyses
of studies across six continents. International Journal of
Epidemiology, 43(5), pp.1542–1562.
https://doi.org/10.1093/ije/dyu094

9. The Menopause Charity, 2023. Menopause and stress.
[online] Available at:
https://www.themenopausecharity.org/2023/04/04/menop
ause-and-stress/ [Accessed 2 April 2025].

Chapter 3

1. Adawi, M. et al. (2019). The impact of intermittent fasting
(Ramadan fasting) on psoriatic arthritis disease activity,
enthesitis, and dactylitis: a multicentre study. Nutrients,
11(3), p.601. Available at:
https://doi.org/10.3390/nu11030601

2. Chedraui, P. et al. (2013). Phytoestrogens and their effect on
menopausal symptoms. Gynecological Endocrinology, 29(1),
pp.1–6. Available at:
https://doi.org/10.3109/09513590.2012.705381

3. Chedraui, P. et al. (2013). Efficacy of phytoestrogens for
menopausal symptoms: a meta-analysis and systematic
review. Climacteric, 16(1), pp.104–118. Available at:
https://doi.org/10.3109/13697137.2012.731559

4. Erdélyi, A. et al. (2024). The importance of nutrition in menopause and perimenopause—A review. Nutrients, 16(1), p.27. Available at: https://doi.org/10.3390/nu16010027

5. Gottfried, S. (2021). Women, Food, and Hormones. New York: HarperCollins. Available at: https://www.amazon.com/Women-Food-Hormones-Hormonal-Yourself/dp/0358345413

6. Llaneza, P. et al. (2012). Mediterranean diet and health outcomes in the perimenopause. Climacteric, 15(5), pp.522–529. Available at: https://doi.org/10.3109/13697137.2012.658465

7. Maloh, J. et al. (2023). The effects of a fasting mimicking diet on skin hydration, skin texture, and skin assessment: a randomized controlled trial. Journal of Clinical Medicine, 12(5), p.1710. Available at: https://doi.org/10.3390/jcm12051710

8. Pelz, M. (2022). Fast Like a Girl: A Woman's Guide to Using the Healing Power of Fasting to Burn Fat, Boost Energy, and Balance Hormones. Carlsbad, CA: Hay House. Available at: https://www.drmindypelz.com/fast-like-a-girl/

9. Stanisławska, M. et al. (2014). The severity of depressive symptoms vs. serum Mg and Zn levels in postmenopausal women. Biological Trace Element Research, 157(1), pp.30–35. Available at: https://doi.org/10.1007/s12011-013-9866-6

10. Tarleton, E.K. et al. (2017). Role of magnesium supplementation in the treatment of depression: a

randomized clinical trial. PLOS ONE, 12(6), p.e0180067.
Available at: https://doi.org/10.1371/journal.pone.0180067

11. Yurko-Mauro, K. et al. (2010). Beneficial effects of
docosahexaenoic acid on cognition in age-related cognitive
decline. Alzheimer's & Dementia, 6(6), pp.456–464.
Available at: https://doi.org/10.1016/j.jalz.2010.01.013

12. ZOE (2021). The truth about menopause supplements.
ZOE Science & Nutrition. Available at:

https://zoe.com/learn/podcast-menopause-supplements

Chapter 4

1. Arabpour-Dahoue, M., Mohammadzadeh, E., Avan, A.,
Nezafati, P., Nasrfard, S., Ghazizadeh, H., Mehramiz, M.,
Safarian, M., Nematy, M., Jarahi, L., Ferns, G.A., Norouzy, A.
& Ghayour-Mobarhan, M., 2019. Leptin level decreases after
treatment with the combination of Radiofrequency and
Ultrasound cavitation in response to the reduction in adiposity.
Diabetes & Metabolic Syndrome: Clinical Research & Reviews,
13(2), pp.1137–1140. Available at:
https://pubmed.ncbi.nlm.nih.gov/31336456/

2. Coiante, E., Pensato, R., Hadji, I. et al., 2023. Assessment of the
Efficacy of Cryolipolysis on Abdominal Fat Deposits: A
Prospective Study. Aesthetic Plastic Surgery, 47, pp.2679–2686.
Available at: https://link.springer.com/article/10.1007/s00266-
023-03369-0

3. Deng, X., Zhang, N. & Wang, Q. et al., 2023. Theabrownin of

raw and ripened pu-erh tea varies in the alleviation of HFD-induced obesity via the regulation of gut microbiota. European Journal of Nutrition, 62, pp.2177–2194. Available at: https://doi.org/10.1007/s00394-023-03089-w

4. Erdélyi, A., Pálfi, E., Tűű, L., Nas, K., Szűcs, Z., Török, M., Jakab, A. & Várbíró, S., 2024. The Importance of Nutrition in Menopause and Perimenopause—A Review. Nutrients, 16(1), p.27. Available at: https://www.mdpi.com/2072-6643/16/1/27

5. Fenton, A., 2021. Weight, Shape, and Body Composition Changes at Menopause. Journal of Midlife Health, 12(3), pp.187–192. Available at: https://www.ncbi.nlm.nih.gov/pmc/articles/PMC8569454/

6. Fonseca, V.M., Campos, P.S., Certo, T.F. et al., 2018. Efficacy and safety of noninvasive focused ultrasound for treatment of subcutaneous adiposity in healthy women. Journal of Cosmetic and Laser Therapy, 20(6), pp.341–350. Available at: https://pubmed.ncbi.nlm.nih.gov/30285509/

7. Hurtado, M.D., Saadedine, M., Kapoor, E. et al., 2024. Weight Gain in Midlife Women. Current Obesity Reports, 13, pp.352–363. Available at: https://link.springer.com/article/10.1007/s13679-024-00555-2

8. Jewell, M.L., Weiss, R.A., Baxter, R.A. et al., 2012. Safety and Tolerability of High-Intensity Focused Ultrasonography for Noninvasive Body Sculpting: 24-Week Data From a Randomized, Sham-Controlled Study. Aesthetic Surgery Journal, 32(7), pp.868–876. Available at:

https://doi.org/10.1177/1090820X12455190

9. Kiedrowicz, M., Duchnik, E., Wesołowska, J. et al., 2022. Early and Long-Term Effects of Abdominal Fat Reduction Using Ultrasound and Radiofrequency Treatments. Nutrients, 14(17), p.3498. Available at: https://www.ncbi.nlm.nih.gov/pmc/articles/PMC9459719/

10. Knight, M.G., Anekwe, C., Washington, K. et al., 2021. Weight regulation in menopause. Menopause, 28(8), pp.960–965. Available at: https://www.ncbi.nlm.nih.gov/pmc/articles/PMC8373626/

11. Kou, X., Li, W., Meng, Q. et al., 2024. Citrus Pu-erh tea extract intake before or after lipolysis in simulated digestion reduces the release of free fatty acids. Food Measurement and Characterization, 18, pp.3042–3053. Available at: https://doi.org/10.1007/s11694-024-02385-1

12. Krueger, N., Mai, S.V., Luebberding, S. & Sadick, N.S., 2014. Cryolipolysis for noninvasive body contouring: clinical efficacy and patient satisfaction. Clinical, Cosmetic and Investigational Dermatology, 7, pp.201–205. Available at: https://www.ncbi.nlm.nih.gov/pmc/articles/PMC4079633/

13. Legrand, F.D., Dugué, B., Costello, J. et al., 2023. Evaluating safety risks of whole-body cryotherapy/cryostimulation (WBC): a scoping review from an international consortium. European Journal of Medical Research, 28, p.387. Available at: https://link.springer.com/article/10.1186/s40001-023-01385-z

14. Mark, L.J. et al., 2022. Whole-body cryostimulation in obesity: A scoping review. Journal of Thermal Biology, 106, p.103250.

Available at:

https://www.sciencedirect.com/science/article/pii/S03064565 22000651

15. Melo, A., Moreira, J., Noites, A. et al., 2013. Clay body wrap with microcurrent: Effects in central adiposity. Applied Clay Science, 80-81, pp.140–146. Available at: https://www.researchgate.net/publication/273624336

16. Nojomi, M. et al., 2016. Health technology assessment of non-invasive interventions for weight loss and body shape in Iran. Medical Journal of the Islamic Republic of Iran, 30, p.348. Available at: https://pubmed.ncbi.nlm.nih.gov/27390717/

17. Sharma, N., Chahal, A., Balasubramanian, K. et al., 2023. Effects of resistance training on muscular strength, endurance, body composition and functional performance among sarcopenic patients: a systematic review. Journal of Diabetes & Metabolic Disorders, 22, pp.1053–1071. Available at: https://doi.org/10.1007/s40200-023-01283-5

18. Shin, J. et al., 2024. Efficacy and Safety of Monopolar Radiofrequency for Tightening the Skin of Aged Faces. Cosmetics, 11(3), p.71. Available at: https://www.mdpi.com/2079-9284/11/3/71

19. Silva, T.R., Oppermann, K., Reis, F.M. & Spritzer, P.M., 2021. Nutrition in Menopausal Women: A Narrative Review. Nutrients, 13(7), p.2149. Available at: https://www.ncbi.nlm.nih.gov/pmc/articles/PMC8308420/

20. Simpson, S.J., Raubenheimer, D., Black, K.I. & Conigrave, A.D., 2022. Weight gain during the menopause transition:

Evidence for a mechanism dependent on protein leverage. BJOG: An International Journal of Obstetrics & Gynaecology, Available at: https://obgyn.onlinelibrary.wiley.com/doi/10.1111/1471-0528.17290

21. The British Menopause Society (BMS), 2023. Nutrition and Weight Gain. Available at: https://thebms.org.uk/wp-content/uploads/2023/06/19-BMS-TfC-Menopause-Nutrition-and-Weight-Gain-JUNE2023-A.pdf

22. U.S. National Institute on Aging (NIA), n.d. How can strength training build healthier bodies as we age? Available at: https://www.nia.nih.gov/news/how-can-strength-training-build-healthier-bodies-we-age

23. Zhou, X., et al., 2020. Hypothalamic oestrogen receptor alpha establishes a sexually dimorphic regulatory node of energy expenditure. Nature Metabolism, 2, pp.351–363. Available at: https://www.nature.com/articles/s42255-020-0189-6

Chapter 5

1. Baker, F.C., Lampio, L., Saaresranta, T. & Polo-Kantola, P., 2018. Sleep and sleep disorders in the menopausal transition. Sleep Medicine Clinics, 13(3), pp.443–456. https://www.ncbi.nlm.nih.gov/pmc/articles/PMC6092036/

2. Chien, L.W., Cheng, S.L. & Liu, C.F., 2012. The effect of lavender aromatherapy on autonomic nervous system in midlife women with insomnia. Evidence-Based Complementary and Alternative Medicine, 2012, p.740813.

https://doi.org/10.1155/2012/740813

3. Gharahdaghi, N., Phillips, B.E., Szewczyk, N.J., Smith, K., Wilkinson, D.J. & Atherton, P.J., 2021. Links between testosterone, oestrogen, and the growth hormone/insulin-like growth factor axis and resistance exercise muscle adaptations. Frontiers in Physiology, 11, p.621226. https://www.ncbi.nlm.nih.gov/pmc/articles/PMC7844366/

4. Hachul, H., Brandão, L.C. & D'Almeida, V., 2005. Effects of light therapy on sleep, mood, and temperature in women with menopausal symptoms: A pilot study. Menopause, 12(6), pp.699–705. https://doi.org/10.1097/01.gme.0000179042.73741.7e

5. Harlow, S.D., Elliott, M.R. & Bromberger, J.T., 2018. The dynamics of stress and fatigue across menopause. Psychosomatic Medicine, 80(5), pp.497–505. https://doi.org/10.1097/PSY.0000000000000584

6. Huang, M.I., Yang, Y.C. & Chen, S.C., 2010. The effectiveness of aromatherapy massage on relieving pain in patients with osteoarthritis of the knee: A randomized controlled trial. Journal of Nursing Research, 18(3), pp.164–173. https://doi.org/10.1097/JNR.0b013e3181eda1b8

7. Kanji, G., Weatherall, M., Peter, R., Purdie, G. & Page, R., 2015. Efficacy of regular sauna bathing for chronic tension-type headache: a randomized controlled study. Journal of Alternative and Complementary Medicine, 21(2), pp.103–109. https://pubmed.ncbi.nlm.nih.gov/25636135/

8. Krajewska-Kułak, E. & Sobolewski, M., 2020. The effect of

foot reflexology on the quality of sleep and fatigue in postmenopausal women: A randomized controlled trial. Complementary Therapies in Medicine, 52, p.102452. https://doi.org/10.1016/j.ctim.2020.102452

9. Laukkanen, J.A., Laukkanen, T. & Kunutsor, S.K., 2018. Cardiovascular and other health benefits of sauna bathing: A review of the evidence. Mayo Clinic Proceedings, 93(8), pp.1111–1121. https://pubmed.ncbi.nlm.nih.gov/30077204/

10. Lee, M.S., Choi, T.Y. & Shin, B.C., 2016. Effect of Gua Sha therapy on perimenopausal syndrome: A systematic review and meta-analysis of randomized controlled trials. Maturitas, 92, pp.55–59. https://pubmed.ncbi.nlm.nih.gov/29705467/

11. Shams, T. & Setia, M.S., 2007. Efficacy of aromatherapy in the treatment of postoperative nausea and vomiting: A systematic review. Journal of Clinical Anesthesia, 19(8), pp.627–631. https://doi.org/10.1016/j.jclinane.2007.07.008

12. Shin, Y.H., Lee, M.K. & Lee, J.Y., 2016. Effect of aromatherapy on sleep quality and anxiety of patients. Journal of Korean Academy of Nursing, 46(5), pp.629–638. https://doi.org/10.4040/jkan.2016.46.5.629

13. Shinohara, K., Kodama, A. & Sasaki, K., 2017. Effects of simplified lymph drainage on the body: in females with menopausal symptoms. Journal of Physical Therapy Science, 29(2), pp.211–214. https://doi.org/10.1589/jpts.29.211

14. Soejima, U., Munemoto, T., Masuda, A., Uwatoko, Y., Miyata, M. & Tei, C., 2015. Effects of Waon therapy on

chronic fatigue syndrome: A pilot study. Internal Medicine, 54(3), pp.333–338. https://www.jstage.jst.go.jp/article/internalmedicine/54/3/54_54.3042/_article

15. Schwerd, S. and Schulte, A., 2024. Evaluating Blink Rate as a Dynamic Indicator of Mental Workload in a Flight Simulator. Proceedings of the 19th International Joint Conference on Computer Vision, Imaging and Computer Graphics Theory and Applications (VISIGRAPP 2024), pp.362–368. https://doi.org/10.5220/0012319100003660

16. Stone, M.H., Hornsby, W.G., Mizuguchi, S., Sato, K., Gahreman, D., Duca, M., Carroll, K.M., Ramsey, M.W., Stone, M.E., Pierce, K.C., et al., 2024. The use of free weight squats in sports: A narrative review—terminology and biomechanics. Applied Sciences, 14(5), p.1977. https://doi.org/10.3390/app14051977

17. Xu, Y. & López, M., 2018. Central regulation of energy metabolism by estrogens. Molecular Metabolism, 15, pp.104–115. https://pubmed.ncbi.nlm.nih.gov/29886181/

18. Yeh, M.L. & Chung, Y.C., 2008. The effect of auricular acupressure on menopausal hot flush and insomnia: A randomized controlled trial. Journal of Advanced Nursing, 61(4), pp.451–460. https://doi.org/10.1111/j.1365-2648.2007.04509.x

Chapter 6

1. Addanki, S., Patel, K., Patel, L., Smith, B., Patel, P., Uppalapati, S., & Nathanson, L., 2024. Thyroid Function and Sleep Patterns: A Systematic Review. Cureus, 16(6), p.e63447. https://doi.org/10.7759/cureus.63447

2. Ahmady, F., Niknami, M. & Khalesi, Z.B., 2022. Quality of sleep in women with menopause and its related factors. Sleep Science, 15(Spec 1), pp.209–214. https://doi.org/10.5935/1984-0063.20220021

3. Beroukhim, G., Esencan, E. & Seifer, D.B., 2022. Impact of sleep patterns upon female neuroendocrinology and reproductive outcomes: a comprehensive review. Reproductive Biology and Endocrinology, 20(16). https://doi.org/10.1186/s12958-022-00889-3

4. Binks, H., Vincent, G.E., Gupta, C., Irwin, C. & Khalesi, S., 2020. Effects of Diet on Sleep: A Narrative Review. Nutrients, 12(4), p.936. https://doi.org/10.3390/nu12040936

5. Cattani, D., Pierozan, P., Zamoner, A., Brittebo, E. & Karlsson, O., 2023. Long-term effects of perinatal exposure to a glyphosate-based herbicide on melatonin levels and oxidative brain damage in adult male rats. Antioxidants, 12(10), p.1825. https://doi.org/10.3390/antiox12101825

6. Darwall-Smith, H., 2022. How to Be Awake (So You Can Sleep Through the Night). London: Penguin Life.

7. Dabrowska-Galas, M. & Dabrowska, J., 2021. Physical activity improves sleep quality in women. Ginekologia

Polska, 92(7), pp.487–490.
https://doi.org/10.5603/GP.a2020.0172

8. Dorsey, A., de Lecea, L. & Jennings, K.J., 2021. Neurobiological and hormonal mechanisms regulating women's sleep. Frontiers in Neuroscience, 14, p.625397. https://doi.org/10.3389/fnins.2020.625397

9. Fatemeh, G., Sajjad, M., Niloufar, R., Neda, S., Leila, S. & Khadijeh, M., 2022. Effect of melatonin supplementation on sleep quality: a systematic review and meta-analysis of randomized controlled trials. Journal of Neurology, 269(1), pp.205–216. https://doi.org/10.1007/s00415-020-10381-w

10. Frank, S., Gonzalez, K., Lee-Ang, L., Young, M.C., Tamez, M. & Mattei, J., 2017. Diet and sleep physiology: public health and clinical implications. Frontiers in Neurology, 8, p.393. https://doi.org/10.3389/fneur.2017.00393

11. Hirokawa, K., Nishimoto, T. & Taniguchi, T., 2012. Effects of lavender aroma on sleep quality in healthy Japanese students. Perceptual and Motor Skills, 114(1), pp.111–122. https://doi.org/10.2466/13.15.PMS.114.1.111-122

12. Kravitz, H.M., Kazlauskaite, R. & Joffe, H., 2018. Sleep, health, and metabolism in midlife women and menopause: Food for thought. Obstetrics and Gynecology Clinics of North America, 45(4), pp.679–694. https://doi.org/10.1016/j.ogc.2018.07.008

13. Lewith, G.T., Godfrey, A.D. & Prescott, P., 2005. A single-blinded, randomized pilot study evaluating the aroma of Lavandula angustifolia as a treatment for mild insomnia.

Journal of Alternative and Complementary Medicine, 11(4), pp.631–637. https://doi.org/10.1089/acm.2005.11.631

14. Maki, P.M., Panay, N. & Simon, J.A., 2024. Sleep disturbance associated with the menopause. Menopause, 31(8), pp.724–733. https://doi.org/10.1097/GME.0000000000002386

15. Mehta, N., Shafi, F. & Bhat, A., 2015. Unique aspects of sleep in women. Missouri Medicine, 112(6), pp.430–434. https://www.ncbi.nlm.nih.gov/pmc/articles/PMC6168103/

16. Mohan, M.E., Thomas, J.V., Mohan, M.C., Das, S.S., Prabhakaran, P. & Pulikkaparambil Sasidharan, B.C., 2023. A proprietary black cumin oil extract (Nigella sativa) (BlaQmax®) modulates stress-sleep-immunity axis safely: Randomized double-blind placebo-controlled study. Frontiers in Nutrition, 10, p.1152680. https://doi.org/10.3389/fnut.2023.1152680

17. Salari, N., Hasheminezhad, R., Hosseinian-Far, A. et al., 2023. Global prevalence of sleep disorders during menopause: a meta-analysis. Sleep and Breathing, 27, pp.1883–1897. https://doi.org/10.1007/s11325-023-02793-5

18. Srivastava, J.K., Shankar, E. & Gupta, S., 2010. Chamomile: a herbal medicine of the past with bright future. Molecular Medicine Reports, 3(6), pp.895–901. https://doi.org/10.3892/mmr.2010.377

19. Hussain, D.A.S. & Hussain, M.M., 2016. Nigella sativa (black seed) is an effective herbal remedy for every disease except

death – a Prophetic statement which modern scientists confirm unanimously: A review. Advancement in Medicinal Plant Research, 4(2), pp.27–57. https://www.netjournals.org/pdf/AMPR/2016/2/16-008.pdf

20. Hussain, J.N., Greaves, R.F. & Cohen, M.M., 2019. A hot topic for health: results of the Global Sauna Survey. Complementary Therapies in Medicine, 44, pp.223–234. https://doi.org/10.1016/j.ctim.2019.03.012

Chapter 7

1. Alqarni, A., Wen, W., Lam, B.C.P., Crawford, J.D., Sachdev, P.S. & Jiang, J. (2022). Hormonal factors moderate the associations between vascular risk factors and white matter hyperintensities. arXiv preprint arXiv:2205.05876. Available at: https://arxiv.org/abs/2205.05876arXiv

2. Buettner, D. & Skemp, S. (2016). Blue Zones: Lessons from the world's longest lived. American Journal of Lifestyle Medicine, 10(5), pp.318–321. doi:10.1177/1559827616637066.

3. Ciappolino, V., Mazzocchi, A., Enrico, P., Syrén, M.-L., Delvecchio, G., Agostoni, C. & Brambilla, P. (2018). N-3 polyunsaturated fatty acids in menopausal transition: A systematic review of depressive and cognitive disorders with accompanying vasomotor symptoms. International Journal of Molecular Sciences, 19(7), p.1849. doi:10.3390/ijms19071849.

4. Decandia, D., Landolfo, E., Sacchetti, S., Gelfo, F., Petrosini, L. & Cutuli, D. (2022). N-3 PUFA improve emotion and cognition during menopause: A systematic review. Nutrients, 14(9), p.1982. doi:10.3390/nu14091982.

5. Hot Flashes, Mood Swings—More Menopause Symptoms May Be Worse for Brain Health. (2025). Health.com. Available at: https://www.health.com/more-menopause-symptoms-worse-for-brain-health-11693884.Health

6. Karlamangla, A.S., Lachman, M.E., Han, W., Huang, M. & Greendale, G.A. (2017). Evidence for cognitive aging in midlife women: Study of Women's Health Across the Nation. PLOS ONE, 12(1), p.e0169008. doi:10.1371/journal.pone.0169008.

7. Mosconi, L. (2024). Exploring menopause's impact on women's brain health. NeurologyLive. Available at: https://www.neurologylive.com/view/exploring-menopause-impact-women-brain-health-lisa-mosconi.Neurology live

8. Osburn, S.C., Roberson, P.A., Medler, J.A., Shake, J., Arnold, R.D., Alamdari, N., Bucci, L.R., Vance, A., Sharafi, M., Young, K.C. & Roberts, M.D. (2021). Effects of 12-week multivitamin and omega-3 supplementation on micronutrient levels and red blood cell fatty acids in pre-menopausal women. Frontiers in Nutrition, 8, p.610382. doi:10.3389/fnut.2021.610382.

9. Pes, G.M., Dore, M.P., Tsofliou, F. & Poulain, M. (2022). Diet and longevity in the Blue Zones: A set-and-forget issue?

Maturitas, 164, pp.31–37. doi:10.1016/j.maturitas.2022.06.004.

10. Scans Show Brain's Estrogen Activity Changes During Menopause. (2024). Weill Cornell Medicine Newsroom. Available at: https://news.weill.cornell.edu/news/2024/06/scans-show-brains-estrogen-activity-changes-during-menopause.WCM Newsroom

11. Severe Menopause Symptoms May Take Toll on Brain Health. (2024). The Menopause Society. Available at: https://menopause.org/press-releases/severe-menopause-symptoms-may-take-toll-on-brain-health.The Menopause Society

12. Senff, J., Tack, R.W.P., Mallick, A., et al., 2025. Modifiable risk factors for stroke, dementia and late-life depression: a systematic review and DALY-weighted risk factors for a composite outcome. Journal of Neurology, Neurosurgery & Psychiatry, [online] Published Online First: 03 April 2025. Available at: https://doi.org/10.1136/jnnp-2024-334925

13. Turek, J. & Gąsior, Ł. (2023). Estrogen fluctuations during the menopausal transition are a risk factor for depressive disorders. Pharmacological Reports, 75(1), pp.32–43. doi:10.1007/s43440-022-00444-2.

14. Wieser, K. (2025). Hot flashes, mood swings—more menopause symptoms may be worse for brain health. Health.com. Available at: https://www.health.com/more-menopause-symptoms-worse-for-brain-health-

11693884.Health

Chapter 8

1. Basiri, R., Seidu, B. & Cheskin, L.J., 2023. Key Nutrients for Optimal Blood Glucose Control and Mental Health in Individuals with Diabetes: A Review of the Evidence. Nutrients, 15(18), p.3929. https://doi.org/10.3390/nu15183929

2. Basiri, R., Seidu, B. & Rudich, M., 2023. Exploring the Interrelationships between Diabetes, Nutrition, Anxiety, and Depression: Implications for Treatment and Prevention Strategies. Nutrients, 15(19), p.4226. https://doi.org/10.3390/nu15194226

3. Bremner, J.D. et al., 2020. Diet, Stress and Mental Health. Nutrients, 12(8), p.2428. https://doi.org/10.3390/nu12082428

4. Darwin, A.G. et al., 2024. Remotely administered non-deceptive placebos reduce COVID-related stress, anxiety, and depression. Applied Psychology: Health and Well-Being, [online] Available at: https://doi.org/10.1111/aphw.12583

5. Firth, J. et al., 2020. Food and mood: how do diet and nutrition affect mental wellbeing? BMJ, 369, p.m2382. https://doi.org/10.1136/bmj.m2382

6. Friedman, M., 2015. Chemistry, nutrition, and health-promoting properties of Hericium erinaceus (Lion's Mane) mushroom fruiting bodies and mycelia and their bioactive compounds. Journal of Agricultural and Food Chemistry,

63(32), pp.7108–7123.
https://doi.org/10.1021/acs.jafc.5b02914

7. Kerr, P., Kheloui, S. et al., 2020. Allostatic load and women's brain health: A systematic review. Frontiers in Neuroendocrinology, 59, p.100858. https://doi.org/10.1016/j.yfrne.2020.100858

8. Kulkarni J. Perimenopausal depression - an under-recognised entity. Aust Prescr. 2018 Dec;41(6):183-185. doi: 10.18773/austprescr.2018.060. Epub 2018 Dec 3. PMID: 30670885; PMCID: PMC6299176.

9. Lewis, J.E. et al., 2021. The effects of twenty-one nutrients and phytonutrients on cognitive function: A narrative review. Journal of Clinical and Translational Research, 7(4), pp.575–620. https://www.ncbi.nlm.nih.gov/pmc/articles/PMC8445631/

10. Machin, R. et al., 2023. Adaptogenic Botanicals with Emphasis on Rhodiola rosea and Withania somnifera. European Journal of Medicinal Plants, 34, pp.20–39. https://doi.org/10.9734/ejmp/2023/v34i111168

11. Mori, K. et al., 2009. Improving effects of the mushroom Yamabushitake (Hericium erinaceus) on mild cognitive impairment: a double-blind placebo-controlled clinical trial. Phytotherapy Research, 23(3), pp.367–372. https://doi.org/10.1002/ptr.2634

12. Mulhall, S. & Anstey, K., 2018. Prevalence and severity of menopausal symptoms in a population-based sample of midlife women. Innovation in Aging, 2(Suppl 1), p.711.

https://www.ncbi.nlm.nih.gov/pmc/articles/PMC6228576/

13. Oschman, J.L., Chevalier, G. & Brown, R., 2015. The effects of grounding (earthing) on inflammation, the immune response, wound healing, and prevention and treatment of chronic inflammatory and autoimmune diseases. Journal of Inflammation Research, 8, pp.83–96. https://doi.org/10.2147/JIR.S69656

14. Woods, N.F., Mitchell, E.S. & Smith-Dijulio, K., 2009. Cortisol levels during the menopausal transition and early postmenopause: observations from the Seattle Midlife Women's Health Study. Menopause, 16(4), pp.708–718. https://doi.org/10.1097/gme.0b013e318198d6b2

Chapter 9

1. Bradford, L., Fuller, S. & Green, J.W., 2022. The impacts of menopause on cognitive function. Utah Women's Health Review. Available at: https://uwhr.utah.edu/the-impacts-of-menopause-on-cognitive-function/#citation

2. Capel-Alcaraz, A.M., García-López, H., Castro-Sánchez, A.M., Fernández-Sánchez, M. & Lara-Palomo, I.C., 2023. The efficacy of strength exercises for reducing the symptoms of menopause: A systematic review. Journal of Clinical Medicine, 12(2), p.548. https://doi.org/10.3390/jcm12020548

3. González, A., Calfío, C., Churruca, M. et al., 2022. Glucose metabolism and AD: evidence for a potential diabetes type 3. Alzheimer's Research & Therapy, 14, p.56.

https://doi.org/10.1186/s13195-022-00996-8

4. Grizzanti, J., Holtzman, D.M. & Macauley, S.L. et al., 2023. KATP channels are necessary for glucose-dependent increases in amyloid-β and Alzheimer's disease–related pathology. JCI Insight, 8(10), e162454. https://doi.org/10.1172/jci.insight.162454

5. Kemmler, W., Lauber, D., Weineck, J., Hensen, J., Kalender, W. & Engelke, K., 2004. Benefits of 2 years of intense exercise on bone density, physical fitness, and blood lipids in early postmenopausal osteopenic women: Results of the Erlangen Fitness Osteoporosis Prevention Study (EFOPS). Archives of Internal Medicine, 164(10), pp.1084–1091. https://doi.org/10.1001/archinte.164.10.1084

6. Mosconi, L., Rahman, A., Diaz, I. et al., 2018. Increased Alzheimer's risk during the menopause transition: A 3-year longitudinal brain imaging study. PLoS One, 13(12), e0207885. https://doi.org/10.1371/journal.pone.0207885

7. Mosconi, L., Nerattini, M., Matthews, D.C. et al., 2024. In vivo brain oestrogen receptor density by neuroendocrine ageing and relationships with cognition and symptomatology. Scientific Reports, 14, 12680. https://doi.org/10.1038/s41598-024-62820-7

8. Nasir, Y., Hoseinipouya, M.R., Eshaghi, H. et al., 2024. The impact of exercise on growth factors in postmenopausal women: A systematic review and meta-analysis. BMC Women's Health, 24, p.396. https://doi.org/10.1186/s12905-024-03240-7

9. Nguyen, T.T., Ta, Q.T.H., Nguyen, T.K.O., Nguyen, T.T.D. & Van Giau, V., 2020. Type 3 diabetes and its role implications in Alzheimer's disease. International Journal of Molecular Sciences, 21(9), p.3165. https://doi.org/10.3390/ijms21093165

10. Schoenfeld, B.J., Grgic, J., Ogborn, D. & Krieger, J.W., 2017. Strength and hypertrophy adaptations between low- vs. high-load resistance training: A systematic review and meta-analysis. Journal of Strength and Conditioning Research, 31(12), pp.3508–3523. https://doi.org/10.1519/JSC.0000000000002200

11. SpringerLink, 2021. No Time to Lift? Designing time-efficient training programs for strength and hypertrophy: A narrative review. Sports Medicine. https://link.springer.com/article/10.1007/s40279-021-01490-1

12. Woods, N.F., Mitchell, E.S. & Smith-Dijulio, K., 2009. Cortisol levels during the menopausal transition and early postmenopause: Observations from the Seattle Midlife Women's Health Study. Menopause, 16(4), pp.708–718. https://doi.org/10.1097/gme.0b013e318198d6b2

Chapter 10

1. Aukerman, E.L. and Jafferany, M. (2023) 'The psychological consequences of androgenetic alopecia: A systematic review', Journal of Cosmetic Dermatology, 22(1), pp. 89–95. doi: 10.1111/jocd.14983.

2. Barati, M. et al. (2020) 'Collagen supplementation for skin health: A mechanistic systematic review', Journal of Cosmetic Dermatology, 19(12), pp. 2820–2829. doi: 10.1111/jocd.13435.

3. Chessa, M.A. et al. (2020) 'Pathogenesis, clinical signs and treatment recommendations in brittle nails: A review', Dermatology and Therapy, 10(1), pp. 15–27. doi: 10.1007/s13555-019-00338-x.

4. de Miranda, R.B., Weimer, P. and Rossi, R.C. (2021) 'Effects of hydrolyzed collagen supplementation on skin aging: a systematic review and meta-analysis', International Journal of Dermatology, 60(9), pp. 1049–1057. doi: 10.1111/ijd.15518.

5. Ghazizadeh, S. and Nikzad, M. (2019) 'Evening primrose oil in the management of menopausal hot flashes: A systematic review', Journal of Menopausal Medicine, 25(1), pp. 1–7. doi: 10.6118/jmm.19001.

6. Goluch-Koniuszy, Z.S. (2016) 'Nutrition of women with hair loss problem during the period of menopause', Przegląd Menopauzalny, 15(1), pp. 56–61. doi: 10.5114/pm.2016.58776.

7. Katja, Ž. et al. (2024) 'The Effects of Dietary Supplementation with Collagen and Vitamin C and Their Combination with Hyaluronic Acid on Skin Density, Texture and Other Parameters: A Randomised, Double-Blind, Placebo-Controlled Trial', Nutrients, 16(12), p. 1908. doi: 10.3390/nu16121908.

8. Larmo, P.S. et al. (2014) 'Effects of sea buckthorn oil intake

on vaginal atrophy in postmenopausal women: A randomized, double-blind, placebo-controlled study', Maturitas, 79(3), pp. 316–321. doi: 10.1016/j.maturitas.2014.07.003.

9. Liu, T. et al. (2020) 'Recent advances in the anti-aging effects of phytoestrogens on collagen, water content, and oxidative stress', Phytotherapy Research, 34(3), pp. 435–447. doi: 10.1002/ptr.6538.

10. Patel, D.P. et al. (2017) 'A review of the use of biotin for hair loss', Skin Appendage Disorders, 3(3), pp. 166–169. doi: 10.1159/000462981.

11. Piérard-Franchimont, C. and Piérard, G.E. (2013) 'Alterations in hair follicle dynamics in women', BioMed Research International, 2013, Article ID 957432. doi: 10.1155/2013/957432.

12. Pilz, S. et al. (2018) 'Rationale and plan for vitamin D food fortification: A review and guidance paper', Frontiers in Endocrinology, 9, p. 373. doi: 10.3389/fendo.2018.00373.

13. Prager, N. et al. (2002) 'A randomized, double-blind, placebo-controlled trial to determine the effectiveness of botanically derived inhibitors of 5-alpha-reductase in the treatment of androgenetic alopecia', Journal of Alternative and Complementary Medicine, 8(2), pp. 143–152. doi: 10.1089/107555302317371433.

14. Proksch, E. et al. (2014) 'Oral intake of specific bioactive collagen peptides reduces skin wrinkles and increases dermal matrix synthesis', Skin Pharmacology and Physiology, 27(3),

pp. 113–119. doi: 10.1159/000355523.

15. Trost, L.B., Bergfeld, W.F. and Calogeras, E. (2006) 'The diagnosis and treatment of iron deficiency and its potential relationship to hair loss', Journal of the American Academy of Dermatology, 54(5), pp. 824–844. doi: 10.1016/j.jaad.2005.11.1104.

16. Wong, R.C. and Ellis, C.N. (2016) 'Iron deficiency anemia and hair loss: A review', Journal of the American Academy of Dermatology, 74(5), pp. 849–856. doi: 10.1016/j.jaad.2015.11.041.

17. Zouboulis, C.C. et al. (2022) 'Skin, hair and beyond: the impact of menopause', Climacteric, 25(5), pp. 434–442. doi: 10.1080/13697137.2022.2050206.

Chapter 11

1. Buyalskaya, A., Ho, H., Milkman, K.L. and Camerer, C.F. (2023) 'What can machine learning teach us about habit formation? Evidence from exercise and hygiene', Proceedings of the National Academy of Sciences, 120(17), e2216115120. https://doi.org/10.1073/pnas.2216115120

2. Clear, J. (2018) Atomic Habits: An Easy & Proven Way to Build Good Habits & Break Bad Ones. New York: Avery.

3. Fogg, B.J. (2020) Tiny Habits: The Small Changes That Change Everything. Boston: Houghton Mifflin Harcourt.

4. Gardner, B., Lally, P. and Wardle, J. (2012) 'Making health habitual: the psychology of "habit-formation" and general practice', British Journal of General Practice, 62(605), pp.

664–666. https://doi.org/10.3399/bjgp12X659466

5. Gollwitzer, P.M. (1999) 'Implementation intentions: Strong effects of simple plans', American Psychologist, 54(7), pp. 493–503. https://doi.org/10.1037/0003-066X.54.7.493

6. Kwasnicka, D., Dombrowski, S.U., White, M. and Sniehotta, F.F. (2016) 'Theoretical explanations for maintenance of behaviour change: a systematic review of behaviour theories', Health Psychology Review, 10(3), pp. 277–296. https://doi.org/10.1080/17437199.2016.1151372

7. Lally, P., van Jaarsveld, C.H.M., Potts, H.W.W. and Wardle, J. (2010) 'How are habits formed: Modelling habit formation in the real world', European Journal of Social Psychology, 40(6), pp. 998–1009. https://doi.org/10.1002/ejsp.674

8. ScienceDaily (2023) 'What can machine learning teach us about habit formation? Evidence from exercise and hygiene'. Available at: https://www.sciencedaily.com/releases/2023/04/23041715 5750.htm (Accessed: 19 April 2025).

9. Verplanken, B. and Wood, W. (2006) 'Interventions to break and create consumer habits', Journal of Public Policy & Marketing, 25(1), pp. 90–103. https://doi.org/10.1509/jppm.25.1.90

Chapter 12

1. Anderson, D., Seib, C. and Rasmussen, L., 2014. Can physical activity prevent physical and cognitive decline in postmenopausal women? Maturitas, 79(4), pp.386–390.

2. Buyalskaya, A., Ho, H., Milkman, K.L., Li, X., Duckworth, A.L. and Camerer, C.F., 2023. What can machine learning teach us about habit formation? Evidence from exercise and hygiene. Proceedings of the National Academy of Sciences, 120(17), e2216115120. https://doi.org/10.1073/pnas.2216115120

3. Cognitive Problems in Perimenopause: A Review of Recent Evidence, 2023. Menopause: The Journal of The North American Menopause Society, 30(1), pp.1–10. Available at: https://pmc.ncbi.nlm.nih.gov/articles/PMC10842974/ [Accessed 19 Apr. 2025].

4. Effectiveness of lifestyle related interventions to improve quality of life among postmenopausal women, 2023. Journal of Education and Health Promotion, 12(270). Available at: https://journals.lww.com/jehp/fulltext/2023/11270/effectiveness_of_lifestyle_related_interventions.388.aspx [Accessed 19 Apr. 2025].

5. Healthy Aging in Menopause: Prevention of Cognitive Decline and Alzheimer's Disease, 2024. Geriatrics, 4(1), p.7. Available at: https://www.mdpi.com/2673-9488/4/1/7 [Accessed 19 Apr. 2025].

6. Lally, P., van Jaarsveld, C.H.M., Potts, H.W.W. and Wardle, J., 2010. How are habits formed: Modelling habit formation in the real world. European Journal of Social Psychology,

40(6), pp.998–1009. https://doi.org/10.1002/ejsp.674

7. Lifestyle Approaches for Maintaining Optimal Health and Wellness, 2025. The Institute for Functional Medicine. Available at: https://www.ifm.org/articles/perimenopause-lifestyle-approaches-for-maintaining-optimal-health-and-wellness [Accessed 19 Apr. 2025].

8. Promoting good mental health over the menopause transition, 2023. The Lancet, 401(10378), pp.123–125. Available at: https://www.thelancet.com/journals/lancet/article/PIIS014 0-6736(23)02801-5/fulltext [Accessed 19 Apr. 2025].

9. The Importance of Nutrition in Menopause and Perimenopause—A Review, 2024. Nutrients, 16(1), p.123. Available at: https://www.mdpi.com/2072-6643/16/1/123 [Accessed 19 Apr. 2025].

Chapter 13

1. Anderson, D., Seib, C. and Rasmussen, L., 2014. Can physical activity prevent physical and cognitive decline in postmenopausal women? Maturitas, 79(4), pp.386–390.

2. Bromberger, J.T. and Epperson, C.N., 2023. Promoting good mental health over the menopause transition. The Lancet, 401(10378), pp.123–125. Available at: https://www.thelancet.com/journals/lancet/article/PIIS014 0-6736(23)02801-5/fulltext

3. Cauley, J.A., 2015. Bone health during the menopause transition and beyond. Clinical Obstetrics and Gynecology,

58(3), pp.539–556. doi:10.1097/GRF.0000000000000136.

4. Epperson, C.N., Sood, R. and Wisner, K.L., 2023. Cognitive problems in perimenopause: a review of recent evidence. Menopause: The Journal of The North American Menopause Society, 30(1), pp.1–10. Available at: https://pmc.ncbi.nlm.nih.gov/articles/PMC10842974/

5. Garg, R., Sharma, R. and Gupta, R., 2023. Effectiveness of lifestyle related interventions to improve quality of life among postmenopausal women. Journal of Education and Health Promotion, 12(270). Available at: https://journals.lww.com/jehp/fulltext/2023/11270/effecti veness_of_lifestyle_related_interventions.388.aspx

6. Greendale, G.A., Lee, N.P. and Arriola, E.R., 2012. The menopause transition and women's health at midlife: a progress report. Menopause, 19(10), pp.1111–1116. doi:10.1097/GME.0b013e318268f06b.

7. Groeneweg, G., 2024. Healthy aging in menopause: prevention of cognitive decline and Alzheimer's disease. Geriatrics, 4(1), p.7. Available at: https://www.mdpi.com/2673-9488/4/1/7

8. Lally, P., van Jaarsveld, C.H.M., Potts, H.W.W. and Wardle, J., 2010. How are habits formed: modelling habit formation in the real world. European Journal of Social Psychology, 40(6), pp.998–1009. https://doi.org/10.1002/ejsp.674

9. Sacco, R., Mancinelli, R. and Berloco, F., 2024. The importance of nutrition in menopause and perimenopause— A review. Nutrients, 16(1), p.123. Available at:

https://www.mdpi.com/2072-6643/16/1/123

10. Tariq B, Phillips S, Biswakarma R, Talaulikar V, Harper JC. Women's knowledge and attitudes to the menopause: a comparison of women over 40 who were in the perimenopause, post menopause and those not in the peri or post menopause. BMC Womens Health. 2023 Aug 30;23(1):460. doi: 10.1186/s12905-023-02424-x. PMID: 37648988; PMCID: PMC10469514

Printed in Dunstable, United Kingdom

67881416R00245